Praise

for *Penis Exercises*

“Whether you are a beginner that has just found out about natural penis enlargement or an experienced veteran like myself, you are sure to enjoy and learn something from *Penis Exercises* . . . My advice: Get the book. I highly recommend it!"
-A.J. "Big Al" Alfaro, penile coach and author of For Men Only

"I gained over two inches in length and one inch in girth. My girlfriend is amazed and doesn't know what is going on but loves it. She comes all the time now because I can reach places I couldn't before. I only wish I knew about penis enlargement years ago. I thought it wasn't possible without surgery. Now I believe.”
-Chris, a 47-year-old reader

"I just read *Penis Exercises*. My suggestion would be: Get the book. Make it your bible. Follow religiously. Measure today. Measure in 365 days. Don't even consider penis enlargement surgery. A moderately large unit is better than failed surgery."
-A surgeon from Germany

“These exercises changed my life. I don't feel insecure while having sex anymore, and I feel like I have total control of my life. In a little over two months, I gained two centimeters (0.8 inches) in length and also two centimeters in girth. I am amazed. If I can do it, anyone can!”
-Martin, a 23-year-old reader

"You can tell the editors of PEGym.com took the time to cultivate one for the bookshelf. If you're serious about penis enlargement, you NEED this book!"
-David Owen, a reader from Florida

"There's so much more to life and to sex than the size of your penis. . . But, the health of the penis can make or break relationships. This book offers an excellent introduction both to the health and to the enlargement of the penis. It's also interesting that enlargement of the clitoris (the female version of the penis) is a known side effect of some medicines, but doctors seem to be in the dark about the fact that the penis can be enlarged."
-Charles Runels, M.D., Author of Anytime...for as Long as You Want

"For men who hope to have sexual relations with their partners into their 70s, 80s and longer, or for men who wish they weren't already relying on a little blue pill to assure their sexual abilities, *Penis Exercises* has the information you need to transform and revitalize your sex life. With clear and useful instructions, this book will literally put the future of your sex life in your own hands. Thou-sands of men have practiced these exercises to restore and retain – and even improve – their sexual vitality. Now you can, too."
-Carl Anderson, Dr. P.H.

"Having a thorough understanding of the penis exercising basics is a must for anyone looking to walk the proper path towards a healthier, stronger and yes...bigger penis. I got *Penis Exercises* about a year into my journey towards a bigger and healthier penis. Although I was far from a beginner, *Penis Exercises'* combination of thorough explanations with their accompanying pictures did a great job at correcting some flaws in my technique and routine. Ever since then, my PE journey has soared to ever increasing heights. Thanks, PEGym.com!"
-J.R.N., a reader from New York

"If you are interested in this subject, *Penis Exercises* will guide you, save you much the time, expense and frustration that you might otherwise expend researching the various methods. I found myself at an impasse as to how to advance. Luckily, I happened upon *Penis Exercises,* which brought clarity to the subject. Now I am back on path!"
-Thomas Seay, a reader from Palo Alto

"I gained 1.5 inches in length and nearly an inch in girth in roughly a year —putting me at the statistical average. To me, PE is like working out for your body, only for your penis. I feel good when I lift weights and run, and I feel good when I exercise my penis. It is just one facet on my road of self improvement. "
-Gary, a 32-year-old reader from Pennsylvania

"This book is very insightful, clear and concise. It could have been called *The Idiot's Guide to a Bigger and Healthier Penis*, because that is essentially what this book is. It took me every bit of two days to read front to back. I tabbed pages of special importance as well as exercises that are currently in my routine. GREAT READ and GREAT BUY."
-A reader from Texas"

What I like best about the book is . . . the whole damn book! It is easy-to-read, easy on the eyes and the tutorial pictures are clear. Instructions are precise and not quirky."
-A reader from New York

"Finally, another step towards bringing penile exercising to the masses in a positive manner. Major kudos to the PEGym.com!"
-Ben, a reader from Alabama

"To all who have not gotten this book: I highly recommend it! I have now finished reading up to Part 4, and I can't wait to read the rest after I actually finish my first five weeks. The main points I like most about the book are: it is very simple-to-read, very detailed in exercises and routines, and it pretty much has everything that you need in an arms-length to get started."
-A reader from Washington

"Penile exercising has given me a larger, healthier penis. My new penis allows my wife to have harder and stronger climaxes than she ever had before . . . and my erections stay harder and last longer than ever."
-Chuck, a 65-year-old reader from New York

"This book rocks! It is heads above any penis exercising book I have ever seen. Take the best information on all the "penis enlargement" web-sites, add great illustrations, photos, graphs and charts. Organize it into logical chapters and sections, make it super easy-to-understand for beginners and advanced guys alike, and presto . . . you have this book!"
-Alex Lam, a reader from Nebraska

"Due to diabetes, I was only 36 years old when I started experiencing severe erectile dysfunction. Exercising my penis changed all of that. Within months, I was able to consistently obtain healthy, rock-hard erections. I also added over an inch in girth and nearly two inches in length." *-Fredrick Poleking, a reader from California*

"The myth-busting facts are in: exercising the penis properly will make your penis bigger, harder and healthier, and the editors of PEGym.com spell it all out with maturity and a dash of appropriate humor. Whether you are an experienced penis exerciser or just beginning, I believe this book is an absolute must!"
-Jason Anderson, a reader from Illinois

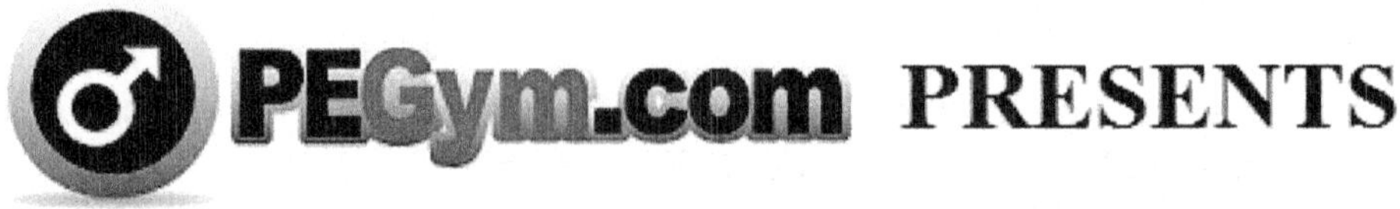

PENIS EXERCISES

A Healthy Book for Enlargement, Enhancement, Hardness, & Health

Editors of PEGYM.COM
Edited by Rob Michaels
Introduction by Richard R. Howard II, Dr. P.H.

PENIS EXERCISES: *A Healthy Book for Enlargement, Enhancement, Hardness, & Health*

Copyright © 2013 Semprove Inc.

To report errors, please email book@pegym.com.

Editor: Kimberly Wylie

Notice of Rights

All rights reserved. No part of this book may be reproduced or transmitted in any form by any means, electronic or mechanical, including photocopying, recording or by any information storage and retrieval system, without written permission from the author, except for the inclusion of brief quotations in a review.

Notice of Trademarks

Trademarks are used throughout this book. Rather than put a trademark symbol in every occurrence of a trademarked name, we instead state that we are using the names in an editorial fashion only and to the benefit of the trademark owner with no intent of infringement of the trademark. No such use or the use of any trade name is intended to convey endorsement or other association with this book.

Dedications

To the men of the PEGym.com community, who are committed to making their sex lives the best they can be.

Penis exercises: a healthy book for enlargement, enhancement, hardness, & health

ISBN-13: 978-0-9887572-0-2

10 9 8 7 6 5 4 3

1. Health. 2. Sexual fitness. 3. Penis enlargement. 4. Self improvement. 5. Penis health.

http://www.PEGym.com

TO THE MEN OF THE PEGYM.COM COMMUNITY,

who are committed to making their sex lives

the best they can be.

Contents

Introduction XII

Part I The Truth Revealed **1**

Chapter 1: MYTH: Penis Enlargement is Impossible 2

Chapter 2: Other Common Penis Myths 5

Chapter 3: What's Average? 13

Chapter 4: Does Size Matter? 16

→ Part I Review 20

Part II The ABCs of Penis Exercising **21**

Chapter 5: Where Do You Stand? 22

Chapter 6: Where Do You Want to Be? Choosing a Goal 25

Chapter 7: The Building Blocks of Penis Exercising 27

Chapter 8: The Basic Principles of Penis Exercising 30

Chapter 9: Principle 1: Obtain Adequate Rest 33

Chapter 10: Principle 2: Gradually Increase the Intensity 35

Chapter 11: Principle 3: Your "Body Clues" 37

Chapter 12: Side Effects are Possible 41

Chapter 13: Look Bigger, Feel Bigger 43

Chapter 14: Pornography and Penis Exercising 47

→ Part II Review 52

Part III The Fundamental Penis Exercises **53**

Chapter 15: The Importance of the Kegel 54

Chapter 16: Kegel Exercises 59

Chapter 17: Kegel Pitfalls 63

Chapter 18: The Importance of Warming Up 65

Chapter 19: Warming Up, It's that Easy 67

Chapter 20: On the Safe Side 73

Chapter 21: Jelqing 75

Chapter 22: Your Erection Level 78

Chapter 23: Jelqing: Step-by-Step 82

Chapter 24: Stretching 88

Chapter 25: Basic Stretching: Step-by-Step 89

Chapter 26: The JAI Stretch: Quick & Easy 93

→ Part III Review 95

Part IV The First 5 Weeks **96**

Chapter 27: Basic Beginner's Routine 97

Chapter 28: Alternative Beginning Routines 100

Chapter 29: Your Unique Goals 106

Chapter 30: Your Unique Penis 108

Chapter 31: Putting the Circle of Gains into Practice 111

Chapter 32: Maximizing Gains 115

Chapter 33: Overcoming Side Effects & Setbacks 122

Chapter 34: The End of the First 5 Weeks 140

→ Part IV Review 142

Part V After the First 5 Weeks **143**

Chapter 35: Advancing 144

Chapter 36: Advanced Exercises 147

Chapter 37: Increasing Intensity of Your Exercises 151

Chapter 38: Basic Advancing Routine 154

Chapter 39: Alternative Advancing Routines 157

Chapter 40: Plateaus and Breaks 165

Chapter 41: Cementing Your Goal 169

→ Part V Review 173

Appendices

Appendix A: 11 Questions Men Ask 174

1. Time is Limited 174
2. Fixing a Penis Curve 175
3. Becoming Multi-Orgasmic 178
4. Erection Difficulties 180
5. Penis Supplements 181
6. Penis Enlargement Pills 183
7. Gaining Troubles 184
8. Penis Enlargement Devices 185
9. Penis Enlargement Surgery 192
10. Increasing Flaccid Size 194
11. Premature Ejaculation 197

Appendix B: The Penis Anatomy 204

Appendix C: Exercise guide & Advanced Exercises 212

Appendix D: Penis Exercising Resources 245

Appendix E: Penis Exercising Success Stories 254
Appendix F: Survey: Ejaculating After Penis Exercise 270
Appendix G: Glossary 272
Afterword 280
Reference Notes 282
Index 288
Acknowledgments 292
Endnote 294

Disclaimer

This is not your average book. There's so much confusion and misunderstanding about the penis today. With the growing popularity of the Internet, you've no doubt seen the penis enlargement advertisements. Just as likely, you've no doubt heard that these advertisements are bogus and penis enlargement is impossible. So where does this leave a man who wants to enlarge and better his penis? Stuck. Confused. Lost.

Be lost, confused, and stuck no more. *Penis Exercises* will change the way you think about penis exercises and penis enlargement. It will change the way you look at your penis. It will change your penis. The information within this book is based on the experiences and reports of thousands of men. Nevertheless, you are using this book at your sole discretion. This book is intended for healthy men over the age of 18. This book is solely for informational and educational purposes and is not medical advice. The publisher, the author, and anyone else who contributed to this book are in no way responsible for what you to do yourself or your penis. Before beginning any exercise program—penile or body—you should consult a physician. The information contained in this book should not be used to diagnose or otherwise treat any illness or health condition.

Penis exercising is not an instantaneous process. It takes time. Any man who decides to exercise his penis in an effort to make it bigger, harder, and healthier must expect to invest time and effort into it. For many men, penis exercises are safer, cheaper, and healthier than prescribing to erection drugs or undertaking penis enlargement surgery. Still, an injury is possible when any exercise is used improperly, including penis exercises (in which an injury can range from a darker penis to complete penile dysfunction). If you engage in the exercises listed in this book, you do so at your own risk.

You should not rush through the exercises in an effort to speed up the process. Many men do, and this is where penis exercises stop becoming healthy and starts becoming dangerous. In the case of penis exercises, less is really more. Doing more than you can handle is a recipe for over-training and often results in temporary erectile dysfunction. This occurs not because the penis is broken, but because it's worn out and needs rest. If you have symptoms of an injury related to penis exercises, see your doctor immediately.

Author's Note

In your hands is a gateway to knowledge that will keep your penis healthy for life. This knowledge doesn't come from just one man—it comes from an entire community. Hundreds of thousands of men ranging from doctors to regular guys have exercised their penis in an effort to make it bigger and harder. These men reside in Internet communities, such as Thunder's Place and The PE Gym, to share their stories and experiences. Without these men, particularly ThunderSS and the many men that make up his place, this book would not be as detailed and precise as it is.

Throughout this book, you will find quotes of these men. Unless otherwise noted, an online alias is used.

To the men of the penis enlargement community: Thank you for sharing your stories. Thank you for your experiences. Most importantly, thank you for your advice.

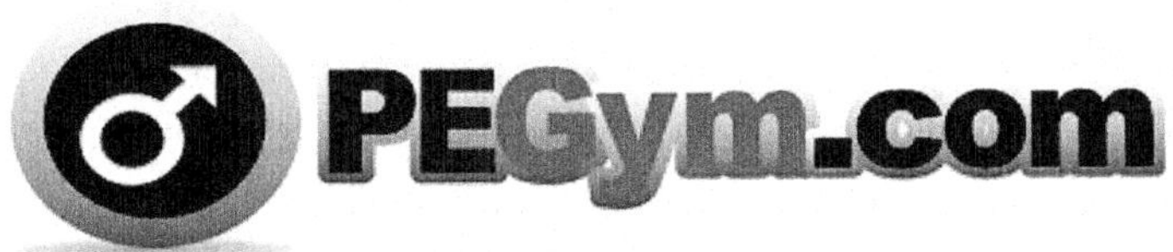

Rob Michaels

Introduction

This book contains insights that may be considered by some, unusual, to others a welcome breakthrough of a subject that many men are keenly interested—improving their penis.

For the individual to achieve wholeness, all aspects of humanity must be presented with a frank and open dialogue that shed light on ideas for self-improvement. Let's start with mythological stories a millennia ago where the concept of physical perfection has its roots. For example, Hercules, in Roman mythology, was noted for his courage and great strength. He symbolized physical perfection. This general stream of consciousness over time ranging from the early Roman Olympics to the present day Olympics gave rise to an evolution of concepts of physical fitness and the attainment of ideal muscularity and athleticism. Particularly over the last century, related areas gained prominence such as body building and aerobic sports leading to the major present day "industry" of physical fitness and health.

Penis Exercises inadvertently asks the question: At what point does the scientific community assert themselves? The classic scientific community seeks strict controlled experimentation with statistically significant results for the validation of a concept. I have found that the historical evolution of a health-related concept often progress along the following time line. Concept development first starts with empirical observation. For example, the sport of bodybuilding came into prominence in the late nineteenth century if not earlier. Men (and women) began lifting crude hand-held weights and soon found that it caused their muscles to grow. As time progressed, there were many pioneers of this field that started to systematize through their publications weight lifting methods and bodybuilding.

The use of weights to stimulate muscle growth became empirically undeniable long before the scientific community subjected it to vigorous experimentation. Yet, now the principle of fitness proliferates enormously, in which every major hospital, city, and town have multiple sports fitness facilities. The long overdue scientific approval on the benefits of health and exercise show how the scientific community can be a lagging participant in inquiry and revelation. It could be said that the same is true for the growth of the supplement industry, which had its humble beginnings in your local pharmacy. Today it has evolved into a billion dollar mega industry including major "health food" chains and supplement outlets. Here too scientific inquiry and "proof" lagged.

Similar to the humble beginning of weightlifting and supplements, the concept of penis health and enlargement has blossomed in recent time. There has historically been a predisposition to suppress the full appreciation of human sexuality and its importance as segments of society have been disinclined to accept human nature. The advent of erectile dysfunction drugs, such as Viagra and others, have catalyzed sexuality awareness and thawed outdated suppression. The billions of dollars in erection drug sales make an irrefutable statement and mandate that sexuality counts and counts in a big way.

Now that sexuality is expressed openly, the time to formulate hypotheses of penis health, strength, and enlargement as additional compelling concepts to the "complete" physical fitness aesthetics paradigm has arrived. The courageous pioneering work in this book seeks to do just that. He has tirelessly acquired a substantial volume of information on this subject and presented it in a logical, sequential way. The book's organization enables you to effectively study and apply point by point these principles, leading to increased health, strength, and size of your most prized organ—the penis.

Richard R. Howard II, Dr. P.H., MS, MPH
(Tulane University Graduate)
Lead Trainer at YourPenisDoctor.com

The Truth Revealed

Part I

In this part you will learn:

- The truth about penis enlargement and penis exercises
- The average penis size is probably much smaller than you think

1

MYTH: Penis Enlargement is Impossible

"Anything is possible. The impossible just takes longer."

– Dan Brown

FACT: Through exercise, penis enlargement is possible.

I will never forget the first lecture I gave on penis enlargement. The audience, a college level sexual education class, refused to believe that the penis can enlarge through exercises. I couldn't blame the class, though. Common knowledge is that men are stuck with the penis they're born with, even though this knowledge is wrong.

Fortunately, the myth that "penis enlargement is impossible" is gradually fading away. More than enough anecdotal evidence has surfaced in the past 10 years to show that, contrary to popular belief, exercising the penis does make it bigger and harder. Penis exercising, as I refer to it, is now widespread on the Web. The Internet provides a vast amount of evidence for penis enlargement. At least 1.3 million men have tried exercising their penis.[1] Many of these men reside in online communities to discuss their experiences and results.

One twenty-year-old reported:[2]

> *When I first started exercising my penis, I was doubtful at best. Since then, my mindset has completely changed. I've been using these exercises for two weeks and I've already gained a quarter inch of length and a quarter inch of girth (in circumference). My flaccid size has also increased by 20 percent!*

A thirty-two-year-old recounted:

> *I have gained over 1.5 inches of length and 0.5 inches of girth in a year. My wife and I both think this is remarkable and still have a hard time believing how much my penis has changed. Even better, I'm much more confident. It's crazy how this one activity—exercising my penis—seems to affect just about everything in my life. Why couldn't I have found out about this stuff 15 years ago?*

And one forty-five-year-old man said:

> *I started exercising my penis because it pained me to think my penis would be small all my life. I put a lot of time into penis exercises, but it was well worth it. After a year and a half, I gained a total of 3 inches in length and 1.5 inches in girth. Believe it or not, penis enlargement really is possible!*

In 2005, I conducted a survey about penis exercises—the first of its kind—in which nearly 1000 men participated. The results showed that the men who exercised their penis for three months or more had gained an average of 1 inch in length and 0.5 inches in girth. Transferring these measurements into volume shows that the men on average increased their penis size by nearly 50 percent.

In *Penis Enlargement Methods*, author Gary Griffin cites a studywith similar success. The study was conducted by Dr. Brian Richards in 1975 and was sent for publication to the British Medical Journal and the British Journal of Sexual Medicine. In the study, thirty men enrolled in a penis enlargement program with exercises similar to the ones found in this book. The program lasted three months. By the study's end, twenty-eight men "demonstrated permanent and verifiable enlargement." The average length increase was 1.125 inches and the average girth increase was 1 inch.

The largest size growth reported to date is by a man who started with 4.5 inches in length and 3.5 inches in girth. In two years, he increased his penis size to 8 inches in length and 5.625 inches in girth. In terms of volume, his penis is nearly five times bigger. Although his results are well ahead of the standard, he's not alone. Countless men have added multiple inches to their penis using the exercises found in this book.

2

Other Common Penis Myths

"All truth passes through three stages. First, it is ridiculed. Second, it is violently opposed. Third, it is accepted as being self-evident."
- Arthur Schopenhauer, philosopher

The belief that penis enlargement is impossible isn't the only myth regarding the penis—there are several more. Many of these myths are part of the overall problem with the current mainstream view of penis exercises. In no small part, these myths play a large role in why society is unaware of the many benefits that exercising the penis provides. It's time to change these false beliefs and put these myths to rest, once and for all.

MYTH: The penis is not a muscle.

FACT: The penis is approximately 50 percent smooth muscle.

"There aren't any penis-building exercises for men because the penis isn't a muscle," argues author Rachel Swift in Satisfaction Guaranteed. Although this is accepted as conventional wisdom by most, it's actually a myth. The penis is roughly half muscle.

This myth has survived for so long because the muscle within the penis isn't your traditional muscle, like your biceps. There are three kinds of muscle: skeletal muscle, which are the muscles you exercise when you go to the gym; cardiac muscle, which is your heart; and smooth muscle, which is found in organs and blood vessels. The penis largely consists of smooth muscle.

All three muscles have their differences, but their structures are essentially alike. Each is made up of proteins, which are vital to all muscle function. Also, both skeletal muscle and smooth muscle grow when placed under stress, such as exercise.[1] One study even showed that injecting skeletal muscle cells into the penis' smooth muscle improved hardness and erection strength, showing just how much the two muscles are alike.[2]

The truth is, smooth muscle is as important to your penis as cardiac muscle is to your heart. "The proper functioning of the smooth muscle is necessary for the normal erection process," says Dr. Michael DiSanto of the University of Pennsylvania. "The smooth muscle in the penis, unlike most other smooth muscle, spends the majority of its time contracted and relaxes only when it receives stimulation." When the smooth muscle relaxes, the penis quickly fills up with blood. Simultaneously, the smooth muscle expands and an erection occurs. In a properly working penis, all of this happens within a matter of seconds.

Every man's penis has a different amount of smooth muscle. Some penises have more than 50 percent smooth muscle; others have less than 30 percent. This difference is a major reason why some men can't get an erection and other men can have an erection for hours on end. "The amount of smooth muscle in the penis is the essential factor that determines a man's ability to achieve normal erections," says urologist Dr. Eric Wespes.

Not surprisingly, the amount of smooth muscle in a man's penis appears to decrease as he ages. In one study published in the *International Journal of Impotence Research*, Dr. Wespes measured the percent of smooth muscle in men of different ages. In his study, the men under forty had an average of 46 percent smooth muscle in their penis; men between forty-one and sixty had 40 percent; and men older than sixty had 35 percent.[3] As men get older, their erections gradually get weaker, and their penis often shrinks in size—largely because of a decrease in penis smooth muscle. Because men have dramatically improved their hardness with the exercises found in this book, it makes sense that penis exercises increases the amount of smooth muscle in the penis—although studies have yet to confirm this. Either way, the penis is indeed part muscle; and like its muscular counterparts, the penis enlarges and hardens when exercised.

MYTH: Erection drugs cure erectile dysfunction.

FACT: Erection drugs are a quick one-night fix, leaving the cause of the problem still there the next day.

Erectile dysfunction—the inability to maintain an erection—is the ultimate sexual stop-sign. It's estimated that roughly 200 million men experience erectile dysfunction, and this figure is expected to be at 322 million by 2025.[4]

Mistakenly, many men who have erectile dysfunction blame it on aging. That's because as a man becomes older, he is educated into believing he needs a little blue pill to maintain a healthy erection. But erection drugs are often unnecessary, and sometimes unleash a whole new set of problems. Pills are not the answer. Pills are a band-aid.

Instead of a drug, most men just need to keep their penis in good physical condition. Studies show that certain penis exercises can boost hardness just as much as erection drugs.[5] And in my survey of nearly 1000 penis exercisers, the majority of the men experienced "stronger and harder erections." Here's what one sixty-two-year-old man said:

> *I started experiencing erectile dysfunction at age fifty-five. Over a period of two years, it got worse and worse. Thankfully, I did some research and learned about penis exercises . . . Now my erections are nearly as hard as they were when I was a teenager!*

The best part? A harder penis often turns into a bigger penis. That's because the more blood that flows to your penis, the more you're going to get out of your erections. In fact, many men report that their first gains are quick and abundant, simply because of better blood flow and a harder penis.

Although there is not an official scientific explanation of how penis exercises boosts erection strength, it no doubt has something to do with increasing the smooth muscle in the penis. Also, a few exercises build stronger pelvic floor muscles, which are the muscles that pump blood into the penis and cause an erection.

MYTH: Penis enlargement is a quick, easy fix.
FACT: Penis enlargement takes time.

Whereas some rumors declare that penis enlargement is impossible, other rumors make penis enlargement out to be a quick overnight fix. This "quick fix" rumor is brought about through all the email spam and penis enlargement advertisements. In many ways, these scam sites are the very reason that penis enlargement is believed to be fake.

"Add two inches to your penis in just two weeks!"

Although gaining two inches is clearly possible, gaining it in two weeks is a different story. In fact, it's close to impossible. Two inches in a year or two is more likely. Exercises don't work overnight. No matter what organ or muscle you exercise—whether it's your penis, your abs, or even your brain—the process of self-improvement always takes time and determination. The good news is that if you give it both of these, you will see results.

How long will it take you to acquire the penis size you want? Here's what the men who took my survey reported:

- It took the majority of the men who gained an inch or less—in length, girth (circumference), or a combination of the two—four months or less to gain it.
- It took the majority of the men who gained between 1.1 and 2 inches—in length, girth, or a combination of the two—anywhere from three to twelve months to gain it.

- It took the majority of the men who gained more than 2 inches—in length, girth, or a combination of the two—more than a year to gain it.

To find more details of how long it took the men to gain, see the Average Gains-Time Assessment in Appendix D: Penis Exercising Resources.

The bottom line: One to two inches is fairly common, and generally takes several months to a year to reach, often more. Three inches is not nearly as common, but several men have obtained this and more; it generally takes at least a year. Four to six inches is not common, but has been reported by a handful of men. Either way, every man is different. Some men gain multiple inches in a few months; other men only gain millimeters in a few years.

Multiple factors determine how quickly you see results, including:

Your goal:

If you just want to be harder, you might accomplish this in just a few weeks. If you want to increase your penis size by 100 percent or more

The Perfect Mindset

Change your mindset from '*now, now, now!*' to '*in time, I'll have the penis size I want.*' Why? Because if you start penis exercising with the mindset of 'now or never,' you will either overtrain or you won't make it past the first two weeks. However, if you start penis exercising with the mindset that it will probably take several months and very likely a year or more to build the penis size you want (depending on your goals), then you will have the stamina to see it to the end. You'll make the most out of penile exercising if you consider it a long-term healthy habit, such as brushing your teeth or hitting the gym.

(in terms of volume), you are going to need a long-term commitment.

How often you exercise:

Sticking to a consistent workout plan is necessary, but penis exercises too much is detrimental and can even stop you from gaining.

How you exercise:

Exercising improperly is the biggest downfall for many men, and some men never gain because of it. You 'll learn how to exercise properly and make the most of your gains in Part II.

Other factors will affect how quickly you see results:

This includes genetics, what kind of exercises you use, what kind of routine you follow, and your dedication.

MYTH: Similar to gym exercising, the gains disappear once you stop performing penis exercises.
FACT: The permanency of penis exercises is different from gym exercising. Penis enlargement is often permanent.

The worst part about going to the gym is that you can spend three years building a perfect chest, and then lose it all by taking a year off. Fortunately, penis exercises are different. Once you stop performing penis exercises, the gains often don 't go away. In fact, some men quit performing penis exercises more than ten years ago and haven 't lost a millimeter.

How is the penis growth permanent? It most likely has something to do with the fact that an erection is actually a light form of penis exercise. The penis, along with the smooth muscle within it, is exercised every time you get an erection. Every time you have sex, masturbate, or have a nocturnal erection (a random erection that takes place during your sleep), you 're exercising. These everyday erections aren 't vigorous enough to enlarge your penis; but they help maintain your new size once you've gained.

Not all gains are permanent, though. Some men lose part of their gains as time goes on. Other men lose all of their gains. This might be because they didn't achieve a sufficient amount of erections. To make your gains more likely to be permanent, you will need to follow a cementing routine—which involves weaning yourself off a penis exercise routine, rather than just quitting abruptly.

MYTH: Penis exercises are dangerous.

FACT: Similar to most exercises, penis exercises are healthy.

Some people think penis exercises are dangerous. It's easy to see why. Several men obtain poor advice on how to properly exercise their penis, and as a result they over-train their penis. You can avoid over-training by following a few simple guidelines, which you'll learn in Part II of this book. But not all men know—or follow—the guidelines of penis exercises.

A poor, yet common belief for some penis exercisers is: If I exercise ten minutes a day and see good results, then exercising sixty minutes a day will provide even quicker results. Penis exercising doesn't work this way, and the extreme stress often results in temporary erectile dysfunction. Fortunately, the penis is a durable organ and the erectile dysfunction almost always clears up in a few days. Nevertheless, when a man goes to a doctor and declares that he hasn't been able to obtain an erection in the last two days, the doctor automatically (and rightfully) blames the penis exercises. And most men won't go to their doctor with the good news.

Exercise, so long as it's safe and not overboard, helps ensure longevity and health. It's no mystery that skeletal muscle and heart muscle need to be continually exercised to stay in good condition. Why would the penis—which is also part muscle—be any different?

Consider this: Your heart's job is to pump blood throughout your body. Anything that makes your heart's job easier and more effective—

such as regular exercise—is healthy. Similarly, your penis' job is to be hard enough to have sex for pleasure, connection, and procreation. Anything that makes your penis' job easier and more effective is also healthy. With that in mind, penis exercises—when done properly—are just as healthy for your penis as running is for your heart.

While writing this book, I talked to hundreds of penis exercisers and read reports of thousands. The large majority of these men reported benefits beyond just a bigger penis. They reported increased hardness, better sex, stronger orgasms, and multiple other benefits that come with having a fit and healthy penis. The list below is just some of the many benefits that penis exercises have delivered to other men:[6]

- A bigger flaccid and erect penis
- Harder and longer-lasting erections
- Stronger orgasms
- Multiple orgasms
- Prolonged sex
- Greater intensity in ejaculation
- Larger ejaculation volume
- Further "shooting distance" when ejaculating
- A healthier prostate, which possibly reduces the risk of prostate cancer and other prostate-related diseases
- Greater confidence
- Greater sex drive
- Reduced or eliminated penis curve
- Increased pleasure for both the penis exerciser and his partner
- An overall better sexual experience
- An overall healthier penis and penile vascular system

You will experience many of these benefits as well. If you follow the guidelines properly, give it time, and use good judgment, you'll be on the safest track to not only a bigger penis, but a healthier one too.

3

What's Average?

"Hell, even a 747 looks small if it lands in the Grand Canyon."

—Tom Arnold in response to his ex wife, Roseanne,

who declared he had a small penis.

Before you start performing penis exercises for the wrong reason, you should know that the average penis size is often misunderstood. Many men who have an average-size penis mistakenly believe they are small. Whether it is because of a comment that a partner made, or the fact that another man in the locker room is bigger than them, a lot of guys think they're smaller than they really are.

Pornography adds to this smaller-than-average mindset. In the porno industry, men are often hired for their well-endowed organs. And for many men, the penis in Black Cock Down or Saving Ryan's Privates is the only other erect penis they have to compare too—which is an unrealistic picture of what is average. To get a better understanding of what average is and where you stand, let's sum up two leading studies conducted on penis size.

The Kinsey Study

Alfred Kinsey is often thought of as the father of modern day sexology. His infamous Kinsey Reports, which were written during the 1940's and 50's, are believed to have played a huge role in triggering the sexual revolution. The following is a summary of a Kinsey Report conducted on penis size in 1948. Even after 60 years, it's still the most popular study on penis size.[1]

The method:

A group of 3,500 college males were sent a postcard in the mail. The men were instructed to measure themselves. For length, each male held the postcard to his pubic bone and marked the tip of his penis on the card.

The average results:

Erect penis length: 6.21 inches
Erect penis girth (circumference): 4.85 inches
Flaccid length: 3.89 inches
Flaccid girth: 3.75 inches

The Lifestyle Survey

Kinsey's method was not completely scientifically accurate (what college student wouldn't fudge a few centimeters for the sake of pride?). As expected, this has caused several debates over the results. Here's a study that is most likely closer to the true average. It was conducted in 2001 by Lifestyles Condom Company. [2]

The method:

300 males were measured in Cancun, Mexico by a doctor and a team of nurses. Because the men did not measure themselves, this study is considered one of the most reliable reports on penis size.

The average results:

Erect penis length: 5.88 inches
Erect penis girth (circumference): 4.97 inches

And the Average is . . .

These two studies illustrate what many others do: the average erect length is between five and seven inches, typically right around six inches. The average erect girth is roughly five inches. In some studies, the averages are even less.

Nevertheless, these averages are just that—calculated arithmetic means. There's really no telling what the ideal penis size is. Your confidence in yourself and in your body determines how important penis size is to both you and your partner. If you believe your penis is small, then it's small. If you believe your penis is perfect, then it's perfect. But, if you are around five or so inches in both length and girth, then know that you're not small. You're average. And exercising with the mindset that you're too small is not only unhealthy for your confidence, but it's also liable to cause you to try and speed up the penis exercises process—which is a bigger mistake than Mr. Lucky Charms being at the wrong end of his rainbow during a gold rush.

The simple fact that you're reading this book shows that you probably want to be bigger. That's fine—and normal—regardless if you're average or not. Most men who perform penis exercises actually start out around average. In my survey of nearly 1000 penis exercisers, the average starting size was perfectly aligned with the average penis size found in most studies.

4

Does Size Matter?

"Love is very deep, but sex only has to go a few inches."

-Stacy Nelkin

Does size *really* matter?

I've heard many arguments on the topic of penis size and its importance. Some of the arguments include "my best lover had a big penis" stories. Others include catchy clichés—"it's not the size of the wand, but the skill of the magician." The debate over the importance of penis size has led me to one conclusion: for some people, penis size is completely irrelevant. For others, penis size is considerably important.

Without a doubt, size matters to men. We men, by nature, love to compare and compete. We want to be the fastest, the fittest, the tallest, and the greatest. Naturally, this innate competitiveness branches off to penis size. We want to be the biggest too. A penis exerciser I interviewed said it best, "I think most men wish they were bigger. Take me, for instance: I have an average size penis, but average just isn't good enough—especially for the organ that equates to manhood, virility, and life."

Another penis exerciser who uses the online alias Dino9x7 (the 9x7 stands for his goal size) said, "Size matters to me, mostly because I know I can change it. If I couldn't, I would have just went on my happy way and never really thought about it." Like several other men, Dino9x7 exercises his penis for the best reason: himself.

Although penis size matters to most men, it generally matters much less to women. Sure, many women love the way a bigger penis looks and feels (just the way many men love the way big breasts or a big butt looks and feels). But some men largely misunderstand penis size; they believe a big penis is essential to satisfying women.

According to editor-in-chief of *Men's Health,* David Zinczenko, three-quarters of women say they are satisfied with their partner's penis size.[1] "The vast majority of women don't care about penis size," says Michael Castleman, sex educator and author of Great Sex. "Many surveys have asked women what they look for in a man. It's quite a list: kindness, caring, warmth, tenderness, attentiveness, commitment, shared values, a good listener, a sense of humor, someone who makes a decent living and has no serious vices. A huge penis? Doesn't make the list." That's because most women do not need a big penis to be pleased, teased, and sexually satisfied. As one woman I interviewed told me, "A skillful hand and tongue goes a really long way in the bedroom."

What's more, the majority of vaginal nerve endings are within the first two inches of the vagina entrance. That's why many women say size doesn't matter. Nearly any penis, regardless if it's big or small, is able to bring a woman to orgasm—as long as there is enough foreplay, clitoris stimulation, and vaginal penetration. Still not convinced? Keep in mind what Charles Runels, M.D., said in Anytime . . . For as Long as You Want, "Next time you're worried about the size of your penis, remember that some women actually prefer no penis at all."

But, is Bigger Better?

My own story that led to this book started with a woman who was obsessed with penis size and, more importantly, my lack of it. But she was outside of the norm. Penis size isn't a major concern for many women. Yet this still doesn't answer the "other" question: is bigger better? Most women will admit that a man who is caring, loving, and attentive is a much better lover than a pig-headed man with a big penis. But this doesn't necessarily answer the fundamental question: what if a man who was caring, loving, and attentive also has a bigger-than-average penis? Is bigger better in this situation? Depending on several circumstances, it might.

Consider this: in a penis enlargement study conducted by Dr. Brian Richards in 1975, thirty men enlisted to do penis exercises for three months. Prior to the study, the wives and girlfriends were interviewed about their thoughts on penis size. Richards indicated, "For the most part they expressed unconcern and lack of enthusiasm about penis size."

However, when Richards and his team interviewed them after the study—after the men had enlarged their penises by an average of 1.5 inches in length and 1 inch in girth—a large percentage of the women changed their minds about penis size. "Later when the trials were over there was a dramatic increase in those who found penis size interesting and valuable and who declared they were pleased with the increase and the unexpected effects this produced in themselves," said Richards. "At the time I had my doubts about penis size relevance. This, more than anything else, dispelled that misconception."[2]

Time and time again, penis exercisers log into online forums to reveal their experiences with their new penis: the new moans their wives make in the bedroom, the new infatuation that their partner has with their penis, the better sex life that they now have. Is bigger better? Perhaps. But truthfully, this question can't be answered by anyone but you. I suppose in time you'll have your own answer. Eventually, you may be faced with an even bigger question: what's *too big*?"

What's More Important: Girth or Length?

According to Cosmopolitan magazine, "Penis length isn't nearly as important as girth. The wider his package, the better able you are to feel him against your sensitive vagina walls."

The results of a study conducted at the University of Texas-Pan American concur with Cosmo's assessment. The study, which was published in BMC Woman's Health, surveyed 50 women on whether width or length was more important. "A large majority, 45 of 50, said width was more important," says Dr. Russell Eisenman, author of the study. Eisenman also notes, "No females said that they could not tell any difference."

Part I Review

- ✓ In a survey of nearly 1000 men who exercised their penis for three or more months, the average gain was 1 inch in length and 0.5 inches in girth (circumference).
- ✓ Healthy penile smooth muscle is as important for your penis as healthy cardiac muscle is for your heart.
- ✓ The majority of men report that their erections are "stronger and harder" due to penis exercises.
- ✓ Penis exercising doesn't work overnight, and it may take you anywhere from months to years to reach your goal.
- ✓ The gains you make from penis exercises are often permanent; particularly if you follow a cementing routine once you reach your goal.
- ✓ The average penis size is roughly 6 inches in length and 5 inches in girth (circumference).
- ✓ According to editor-in-chief of *Men's Health* David Zinczenko, three-quarters of women say they are satisfied with their partner's penis size.

The ABCs of Penis Exercising

Part II

In this part you will learn:

- Why measuring is important and the proper way to measure
- A basic overview of penis exercises
- The important principles of penis exercises
- The common side effects to look out for
- 8 ways to make your penis look bigger right away

5

Where Do You Stand?

Measuring

An important part of penis exercises is monitoring your progress. To do that, you'll need to measure. Measuring is naturally important because it allows you to see if you are gaining; and if you aren't gaining, you know you need to change something. Measuring also allows you to know where you are and, more importantly, where you want to be (more on this in the next chapter). Many men also find that measuring motivates them with every gain they make.

How often you measure is your decision. The more often you measure, the easier you'll find it to track your progress and pay attention to your "body clues" (more on these later). Don't, however, get into the habit of measuring everyday looking for a half-inch gain.

Measuring

You'll want to measure two areas: erect length and erect girth. You can also choose to measure flaccid length and flaccid girth if you desire a bigger flaccid penis. To measure, you'll need two items:

- Soft vinyl measuring tape or a piece of string
- Straight edge ruler

Measure Exactly the Same Way Each Time

Consistency is the most important part of measuring. If you aren't consistent, you could fool yourself into thinking you are gaining when you aren't. That's because you can easily gain an extra inch on the ruler by measuring a different way. To consistently monitor your progress, use the same measuring technique each time you measure. For example, if you measure sitting down the first time, measure sitting down every time thereafter. If you measure with the ruler pressed into your pubic down the first time, do it again the next.

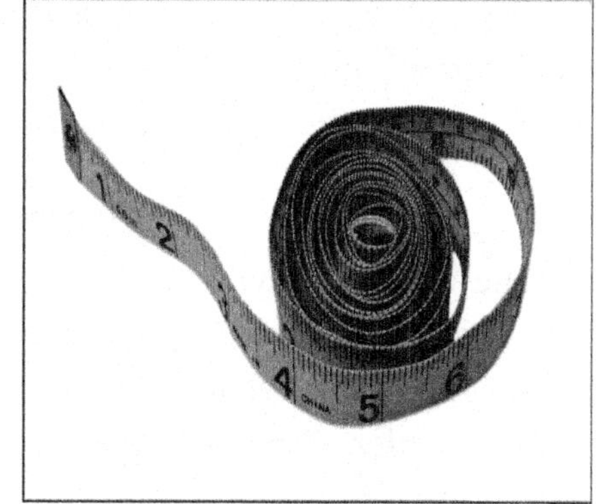

Measuring Tape

Measuring Length

The best way to measure length is with a straightedge ruler. There are two ways to measure erect length:

1. Bone-pressed:

Place the ruler above the penis, firmly press the ruler against your pubic bone, and record your measurement.

2. Non-bone-pressed:

Repeat the same process as above, but don't press the ruler to the pubic bone. The ruler should barely touch the skin of your pubic region.

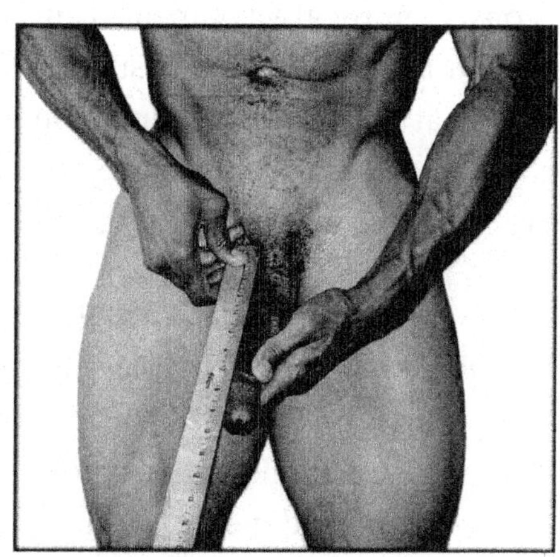

Measuring Non-Bone Pressed

Measuring bone-pressed is well-liked by many penis exercisers because it is more consistent than non-bone-pressed. The reason is that when you measure bone-pressed in the future, you are not able to cheat yourself by pushing the ruler in a little further—the bone will always stop you. Also, several men like the fact that bone-pressed measurements are larger than non bone-pressed. For the best accuracy, measure both.

Measuring Girth: Method 1

The first way to measure erect girth is to use vinyl measuring tape, such as a tailor's tape measure. For this method, wrap the measuring tape fully around your penis once and record the measurement.

Method 2

The second way is to use a piece of string and a ruler. For this method, wrap the string around your penis as you would with a tape measure. Mark the measurement on the string. Take the string and line it up with a ruler. The marking on the string signifies your girth measurement.

Always Measure Girth in the Same Place

Because your penis might be thicker in some places, you'll want to stay consistent by always measuring your girth in the same place. The two most common places to measure girth are the middle of the penis (mid-shaft) and at the thickest point. You can measure both or just one. If you want to be extremely accurate, measure in three different areas: base (where the penis exits the body), mid-shaft, and the head of the penis.

Measuring Flaccid

Obtaining an accurate flaccid measurement is often difficult because flaccid size—the size of your non-erect penis—changes frequently. Temperature, diet, and water intake all have an effect on the size of your flaccid penis. You can, however, obtain a fairly accurate flaccid measurement by using the same methods you used to measure your erect penis. To obtain an accurate flaccid measurement, measure at three separate times, add the measurements up, and divide by three.

6

Where Do You Want to Be? Choosing a Goal

"If you aim for nothing, then you'll hit it every time."

-anonymous

After you're done measuring, you'll want to set a goal.

With penis exercises, like all exercises, a goal is essential to seeing results. In the long run, a goal provides you with daily motivation, which is important because the hardest part of penis exercises is staying committed to a program. Exercising the penis is different from going to the gym. The social aspect isn't the same. You most likely won't have your best friend calling to ask if you want to exercise your penises together. You—and you alone—will be your motivation.

One penis exerciser who uses the online alias Hotwrap describes how a goal impacted his gains: "I've been using penis exercises for 14 years. Only recently have I got results. Why? Because I never set a goal. Since deciding on an achievable goal, I've gained more size than in all the years that went before. All you need to do is decide on an achievable goal.

Faith can make anything happen!"

As you choose a goal, realize that the more specific the goal, the better. Depending on what size you're starting with, and what you want to accomplish, you're goal will most likely vary from the next man's. Here is what other men say about their goal:

- "My penis length is currently 4 inches and my girth is 3.75 inches. My goal is simple: I want to be average. Once I reach 6 inches by 5 inches (length by girth), I will be fully content with my penis size."
- "I'm average in size, and I'd like an extra inch of length and an extra half inch of girth—just enough to put me in the above average range."
- "I've just had my 55th birthday and my erections aren't what they use to be. I chalked it up to aging, but now I know I have control. My goal is to never again have to worry if my penis will be ready to 'play' when the wife and I are ready to."
- "I'm starting out with 7 inches of length and 5 inches of girth. I'm shooting for 8 inches by 6 inches. The wife, on the other hand, wants no more length—just girth."
- "My current measurements are 5.5 inches of length and 4.5 inches of girth—just below average. My goal is to be just above average: 7.5 inches of length and 5.5 inches of girth. So I'm ultimately shooting for extra inch of girth and two inches of length."

An even better way to visualize your goal is to use an object that will allow you to actually see your future size. For example, a common goal is 8 inches in length and 6 inches in girth, which just happens to be a common dildo size. To keep themselves motivated, many men buy a dildo and place it where they see it each and every day. Using an object to actually see your future size is the best way to stay motivated. You don't, however, have to use a dildo. A toilet paper roll, a red bull can, or anything that is close to the size you want will do.

7

The Building Blocks of Penis Exercising

"To build a great house, you must first lay a great foundation."

-fortune cookie

When it comes to exercising your muscles, you lift weights and they grow bigger and harder overtime. The same concept applies to exercising your penis. Instead of lifting weights, however, you 're applying stress in one of two ways: stretching or expanding.

Stretching

Stretching literally involves pulling the penis, albeit gently. Stretches are commonly known as length exercises because they work best for obtaining length. For the first five weeks, you will mainly focus on the basic stretch, which will give your penis an effective workout while also help you become familiar with stretching. As time goes on, you will incorporate advanced stretches into your routine.

Expanding

Expansion exercises are commonly known as girth exercises because they use grips, squeezes, and other methods to obtain girth. Some expansion exercises also help obtain length, such the jelq—which pushes blood throughout your penis. For the first five weeks, the jelq is the only expansion exercise you will use.

One Exception: The Kegel

Although stress is typically applied with your hands, the kegel (pronounced KAY-gul) only requires the will of your mind. That's because the kegel is the only penis exercise that strengthens real skeletal muscles. The kegel is also the most important exercise for any man trying to improve his hardness, his penis, and his sex life.

The Routines

After you learn the exercises, you will put them together into a workout routine. Your first routine will mainly consist of the three fundamental exercises: the basic stretch, the jelq, and the kegel. How often you use these exercises is up to you. Some men workout their penis once every few days; others work it out several days in a row. For your penis to grow, you will most likely need to perform penis exercises at least three days a week, for fifteen minutes or more each day (and increase this overtime). To help direct you, I'll provide you with multiple routines to choose from. Each guides you on when to perform penis exercises, how many reps to do, and when to increase the intensity. You can find many more workout routines at http://www.PEGym.com/routines.

Cementing

Once you reach your goal, your main concern will be keeping your gains. To accomplish this you'll need to follow a cementing routine, in which you'll do light exercises for three months in an effort to make your gains permanent.

Enlargement Devices

As a side note, many men also use devices to enlarge and strengthen their penis. This book focuses primarily on penis exercises with your hands, but in Appendix A you'll find an overview of the common devices under the section "Penis Enlargement Devices." With the possible exception of a penis extender, you should avoid penis enlargement devices until you have been performing penis exercises for at least two to three months.

Penis Exercising Principles

Besides the actual exercises, penis exercises aren't much different from gym exercising. When exercising at the gym, there are a few basic principles that will optimize your results. Many of the same principles apply to penis exercises. You'll learn the important ones over the next few chapters.

8

The Basic Principles of Penis Exercising: The Circle of Gains

Scientists, body builders, and fitness trainers learned long ago that you can't just go to the gym, lift weights, and expect to look like Arnold Schwarzenegger (in his Terminator days). Lifting weights is only half the picture. The other half is doing it correctly and in a smart manner—largely by using a couple of basic principles.

Similar to gym exercising, penis exercises also have principles. Likewise, they are easy to learn and essential to building a better penis. Three principles are absolutely vital to healthy and effective penis exercises, and make up what I call the Circle of Gains.

Principle 1: Obtain Adequate Rest

Similar to exercising your body, for growth to occur, your penis needs time to rest and recover from your workouts.

Principle 2: Gradually Increase the Intensity

Also similar to exercising your body, you'll want to increase the intensity as time goes on. This increase is gradual, not rapid. Increasing the intensity too much too soon is a big pitfall for many beginners.

Principle 3: Pay Attention to Your "Body Clues"

This principle is the most important of the three. It involves paying attention to your penis and how it reacts to the exercises. Your body clues let you know if you are exercising healthfully.

The Importance of The Circle of Gains

While writing this book, I interviewed and read hundreds of reports by penis exercisers—along with their triumphs and their failures. Over the course of nearly two years, I analyzed these men the way an auditor analyzes taxes. I picked and pried until it became ultimately clear that the men who gained big followed these principles. They gave their penis rest, they paid attention to their body, and they continually increased the intensity. Most importantly, they exercised with the mindset that penis health comes first.

At the same time, the men who didn't gain didn't follow these principles. They increased the intensity too fast. They didn't pay attention to their body. They didn't obtain enough rest—largely because they felt it would stop them from gaining. (Ironically, these men probably would have gained if they had just taken enough time off.) Many of these men finally had to stop performing penis exercises out of despair or because they were severely over-training.

The principles that make up the Circle of Gains are so important that you will want a solid idea of what they are before you even learn your first exercise. You'll get a better understanding of these principles once you start performing penis exercises; but for now, know that by following these three principles, you will maximize results and minimize injury. The

Circle of Gains is a combination for success. Make it part of your thinking, and you'll be on the fast track to making your penis bigger, harder, and healthier.

GRADUALLY INCREASE INTENSITY
OBTAIN ADEQUATE REST
GAINS
WATCH BODY CLUES

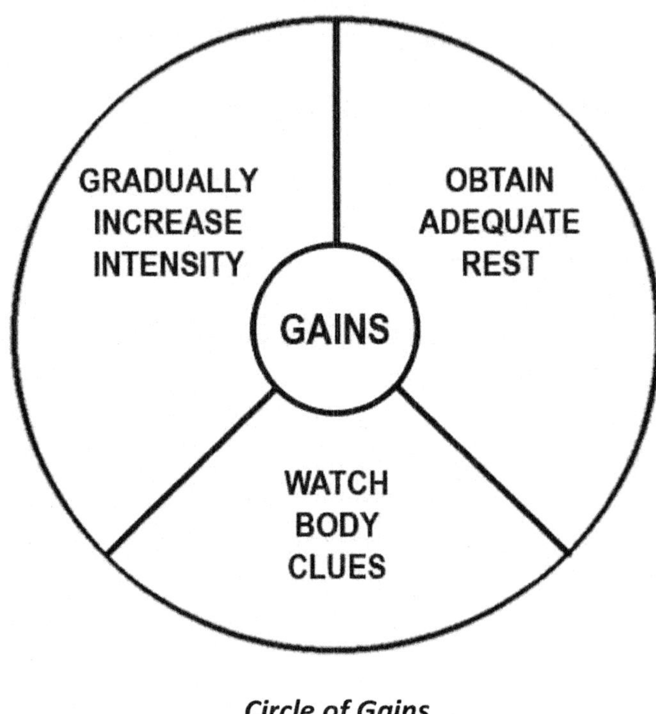

Circle of Gains

9

Principle 1: Obtain Adequate Rest

Like your muscles, your penis needs rest to grow bigger and stronger. Without proper amounts of rest, you 'll over-train your penis, which leads to an effect opposite of your goal—weaker erections and no growth.

Now, some men need more rest than others, and you 'll need less rest as you advance. The amount of rest your penis needs might depend on:

How long you've been performing penis exercises:

The more you perform penis exercises, the more conditioned your penis will become, and the less rest you 'll need. Eventually, after several months, you may be able to exercise your penis six or seven days in a row without any days off. But for the first week, strive to get two days of rest between each penile workout. After that, you can move onto performing penis exercises every other day, and gradually obtain less rest as time goes on.

Your genetics:

Some men can get away with less rest, simply because their penis recovers from the workouts faster.

Other variable factors:

Your age, your diet, and how often you have sex and masturbate (which are both a light form of performing penis exercises).

During your rest days, make sure you are resting. Avoid any of the exercises you'll learn in this book on rest days. Give your penis the time off that it needs to recover and grow.

10

Principle 2: Gradually Increase the Intensity

"Baby steps. One day at a time. One tiny step at a time."

– *Dr. Leo Marvin in What About Bob?*

Let's pretend—for a moment—that you're exercising your biceps. You start out with your max: twelve reps of twenty pounds. As the weeks go on, you become stronger and your max increases. You can technically do twelve reps of thirty pounds, but you don't increase the weight at all. For one reason or another, you stay at twenty pounds, twelve reps.

As a result, you aren't pushing yourself to the max, and your biceps don't enlarge as much as they possibly can. And if you stay at twenty pounds long enough, your biceps will stop growing altogether.

That is because, as Dr. Dan Curtis, M.D., reported, "The amount of stress on the muscle has to be greater than what the muscle typically is subjected to. If you do an activity every day that involves a movement and a weight that does not change, then there is no stimulus for the muscle to grow. But if you increase the amount of stress on the muscle, then there is a stimulus for the muscle to grow."[1]

Although your penis isn't skeletal muscle, it essentially works the same way. It adapts quickly. For growth to occur, your penis needs to be continually challenged with a stimulus that is beyond what it's accustomed to. To do this, you'll have to slowly increase the intensity as time goes on.

In the beginning, you will increase the intensity in one way: by increasing the amount of time spent performing penis exercises. As you progress, you will also increase the intensity in two other ways: by adding advanced exercises and by increasing the intensity of the exercises you are already using, which you'll learn more about in Part V.

A Common Pitfall: Moving Up Too Fast

Although increasing the intensity is essential to continuous growth, increasing the intensity too quickly is the most common downfall for beginners. Many penis exercisers are eager to gain; and as result, they let their ambitions make the decisions. Whatever you do, don't let this happen to you.

Increase the intensity, but do it little by little. The goal is to start out light and condition your penis while you gradually progress. Rushing into high intensity often leads to burning out, to hitting a plateau (where growth stops), or to over-training—all of which can stop growth from occurring.

Never start out with the advanced exercises or attempt to skip steps. Doing so is potentially dangerous. Without proper conditioning, jumping ahead is like having a maximum bench press of 150 pounds and trying to lift 400 pounds.

If you only remember one thing from this chapter, let it be in the beginning, less is more. Penis exercising isn't a competition. It's a union between you and your penis.

11

Principle 3:
Pay Attention to Your "Body Clues"

"Hard is good; Harder is better"

– *Dr. Steven Lamm, The Hardness Factor*

This principle is the most important of the three. That's because your body clues tie everything together. By telling you what's happening to your penis, your body clues help you know when you should rest and when you should increase the intensity.

The body clues were discovered by a chiropractor who uses the online alias Sparkyx. In 2004, Sparkyx discovered something that would change penis exercises forever. He noticed that the penis generally gives off certain healthy clues, such as harder erections, when growth occurs. He also noticed that the penis gives off certain unhealthy clues, such as weaker erections, when no growth occurs.

Group 1: Healthy Body Clues

Healthy clues are a clear sign that you're improving the physical health of your penis. Your main goal is to build a healthy penis first, and a bigger penis second. That's because a healthy penis comes hand in hand with a bigger one. Essentially, if you have all healthy body clues, then you're most likely going to gain.

Group 2: Unhealthy Body Clues

Unhealthy clues are a clear sign of over-training. They're a warning that you're doing something wrong. Think of unhealthy body clues as your penis screaming: "stop, you're doing too much!" In this case, you need to slow down—even if it means doing less exercise than the sample routine recommends. Watching and avoiding these unhealthy body clues will maximize your gains and keep your penis free from injury.

Body Clues Cheat Sheet: A Breakdown of the Common Body Clues	
Healthy:	**Unhealthy:**
• Stronger erections • More frequent erections throughout the night • Waking up with 'morning wood' • Bigger flaccid size • Good flaccid elasticity (a penis that is easier to stretch: not stiff) • Fatigue along the penis (similar to post-gym muscle fatigue; not to be confused with numbness) • Temporary increase in size after a workout • Increase in growth	• Weaker erections • Less frequent erections throughout the night • Absence of 'morning wood' • Smaller flaccid size • Less flaccid elasticity (a penis that does not stretch as easily; stiff) • Lack of sensation or numbness • Bruising • Pain • Temporary decrease in size

The bottom line:

Harder is better. Not only is increased hardness a benefit of penis exercises, it's also a barometer for how well the exercises are working. Strong erections are equivalent to healthy exercising, and are a sign that the exercises are working. Weak erections are equivalent to unhealthy exercising.

Putting it All Together

Paying attention to your body clues is important because every penis responds to the exercises differently. Some men exercise seven days a week without ever over-training; other men over-train with just one day of performing penis exercises. Your body clues are like an atlas on a cross-country vacation. They will guide you on the safest, quickest track to a bigger and healthier penis.

When you experience healthy body clues, it essentially means you're not going overboard and your penis health is improving. Still, there may be times when you experience all healthy body clues but no growth, which indicates that although you are exercising healthfully, you will need to increase the intensity to enlarge your penis. At some point, you may increase the intensity too much and *"over-train"* That's okay, so long as you notice the unhealthy body clues and react accordingly.

When you experience unhealthy body clues, you'll want to stop performing penis exercises and give your penis adequate rest until the

A Healthy Penis

Morning wood—or waking up with an erection—is a good sign that your penis is healthy. In fact, several sexologists use it to determine if erectile dysfunction is psychological or physical. If morning wood is present, the pipes are perfectly healthy and the problem is probably psychological.

unhealthy clues go away. Stopping when you have unhealthy body clues is analogous to pulling over your car when smoke is seeping from the hood. In both cases, something isn't going as planned, and the situation needs to be fixed.

Examples of Men Using their Body Clues

Example 1:

Frank is on his third week of performing penis exercises and he is jelqing for sixteen minutes per workout (four days a week). He experiences three healthy body clues: his penis is growing, his flaccid size is bigger, and he has stronger erections. The healthy body clues signal that Frank's on the right track. To keep the growth coming, Frank gradually continues to increase the intensity. He adds two additional minutes of jelqing each week (so he's jelqing for eighteen minutes the fourth week, twenty minutes the fifth, and so on).

Example 2:

Alex is on his second week of performing penis exercises and he is jelqing for ten minutes per workout (three days a week). During his next workout, Alex rapidly increases the intensity by adding ten extra minutes of jelqing to his routine. After a couple of days, Alex's erections are weak and his flaccid size is smaller than normal—two unhealthy body clues, and an indication that he's over-training To recuperate, Alex stops performing penis exercises and lets his penis rest until his erections return to normal.

12

Side Effects are Possible

We've already talked about all the positive things performing penis exercises can do for you. Now, before you embark into the world of penis exercises, let's talk about the not-so-positive things. If you've ever done an intense workout at the gym, you've probably experienced both positive and negative side effects. You might have felt more energetic—a positive side effect. At the same time, your body might have been sore from such an intense workout—a negative side effect. Both side effects usually don't last long, and don't necessarily happen every time you work out.

The same goes for penis exercises side effects: they are often temporary and you may or may not experience them. Some men never encounter even one side effect. You should also note that most of the negative side effects can be minimized—and even avoided—if you use good judgment and follow the advice in this book. You'll learn how to overcome side effects later on if they occur. In the mean time, you should know what to look out for.

A darker penis:

This side effect can range from your penis being slightly darker in certain spots to your entire penis becoming a darker bronze-like color (many men describe the latter look to be "manlier"). Darkening is the most common side effect and is often associated with intense exercises and over-training It generally takes several months to occur, but this isn't always the case. Just as some people are more prone to bruising, some men are more prone to darkening. Although the darkening effect is often temporary, several penis exercisers have experienced a long-term darkening of the penis.

Stronger and more apparent veins:

For some men, penis exercises cause veins to be more prominent and visible along the penis.

Spots forming along the penis:

Temporary spotting is more common on the glans—the head of the penis—but can happen anywhere along the shaft. The spots are typically red and the size of a pin prick, but they can become larger and darker. Spotting is fairly normal, especially in the beginning. It usually lasts no more than a few days and is generally a sign of using too much intensity.

The doughnut effect:

A temporary swelling of skin near the head of the penis can occur after an intense penile workout. The effect looks like a puffy doughnut formed near the head of your penis and usually lasts no longer than a few hours.

Temporary decrease in size or hardness:

This is a clear indication of over-training When performing penis exercises, think of your penis as you do your muscles: it gets sore and weak when pushed beyond its limits. Again, to avoid this, you'll want to start out light and work your way up.

13

Look Bigger, Feel Bigger

Before you start enlarging your penis with exercises, here are eight ways you can make your penis appear bigger right away. Although the following "quick fixes" don't physically make your penis bigger, they will make it look and feel bigger in uncomfortable situations. Eventually, your penis will be as healthy and as big as you want it and these quick fixes will be irrelevant. In the meantime:

1 - Cut Down on the Pubic Hair

A trimmed pubic region is good for more than stopping your partner from coughing up hairballs. It will also make more of your penis visible. Depending on how long your pubic hair is, you could be covering up to an inch or more of your penis. Note of caution: If you've never trimmed your genital area before, take it slow and use plenty of shaving cream.

2 – Get a Head-On View

In general, the angle we men look at our penis (straight down) doesn't give us a proper idea of how big we really are. To get a better idea, look at yourself naked in the mirror. You may be surprised to find that you're bigger than you think.

3 – Give Your Penis a Light Pull

A gentle tug will often increase your flaccid penis size within a matter of seconds (keyword is gentle, tough guy). Just make sure you pull gently and avoid pulling the head of your penis. Your penis is the most delicate and sensitive part of your body, so treat it that way.

4 – Quit Smoking

Your penis is comparable to a car tire. Instead of filling with air, it fills with blood. When you get an erection, your penis becomes engorged with blood and gets up to seven times bigger. All of this occurs if you have good blood circulation, which smoking puts a big halt to. According to Men's Health Online, "Smoking can shorten your penis by as much as a centimeter. So even if you don't care all that much about your lungs or dying young, spare the little guy."

5 – Don't Urinate

If you are expecting others to see your penis, like in the locker room or at a nudist colony, then don't pee beforehand. When you hold it in for a long period of time, it often leads to inflation in penis size.

6 – Think Stimulating Thoughts

Anything that gets blood flowing to your lower region helps increase the flaccid size of your penis. Be sure, however, that you don't get too much blood flowing at the wrong time, say when you're at the office or a family barbeque.

7 – Think Happy Thoughts

In the movie Magnolia, Tom Cruise plays the role of a seduction guru, during which he tells his audience of groupies to "Respect the cock." And really, Tom Cruise aside, you should respect the cock. Not just any cock. Your cock. Too many men are ashamed of their penis and treat it as if it's their red-headed fifth cousin. No, they don't kick dirt in its face. But they don't treat it with respect either.

Your penis is your penis. Take ownership of your favorite organ. Be proud of what you have and you will gain more than just a few inches —your sexual improvement will expand in miles. Surveys continually show that women want a man who is confident in the bedroom more than they want a man with a big penis.

8 – Lose the Gut

This fix isn't quick, but it's the healthiest fix of them all. As David Zinczenko and Ted Spiker say in their life-changing book, *The Abs Diet*, "When it comes to a man and his privates, fat is his body's side-view mirror. Objects appear smaller than actual size. The length of the average man's penis is about 3 inches flaccid, but the fatter he is, the smaller he'll look. That's because the fat at the base of a man's abdomen covers up the base of his penis. Losing just 15 lbs will add up to half an inch to the length of a man's member. No, Little Elvis is not technically growing, but decreasing the fat that surrounds it will allow all a guy's got to actually show."

Eating healthy and doing regular exercise can also hold erectile dysfunction at bay. A Harvard study that involved more than 30,000 men between the ages of 55 and 90 years showed just how much a healthy lifestyle could help. "The study found that those who regularly exercised typically had a 10-year delay in ED compared with sedentary guys. This amounts to not having to depend on medications or other ED remedies for an additional 10 years, if at all," reports Damon Cozamanis and Marc D. Grobman, authors of *The Penis Diet*.

9 – Take Supplements

There are a variety of effective supplements that can help increase blood flow to your penis, as well as other beneficial effects. Vitamin E has long been associated with increased production of testosterone, as well as improving circulation.[1] Vitamin C improves the lining of the arteries, also increasing blood flow to your penis.[2] The B vitamins have a variety of positive penile effects; however, Vitamin B1 and B3 specifically are known to improve circulation.[3]

14

Pornography and Penis Exercising

Pornography is big business in the United States. There's no business like the porn business! In fact, it has been estimated that pornography is a $10 billion a year industry.

With the increased prevalence of porn, in part thanks to the Internet, there has been much debate over recent years about the use of pornography and whether or not it impairs sexual function. Pornography addiction is a valid concern. However, many feel that pornography can be an enhancement to a normal sex life, as well as a tool to be used with your penis exercising. Let's talk about the pros and cons.

Pornography and Addiction

Before we talk about pornography addiction, it's important to understand the difference between addiction and desire. According to Merriam Webster, an addiction is:

> *(A) compulsive need for and use of a habit-forming substance (as heroin, nicotine, or alcohol) characterized by tolerance and by well-defined physiological symptoms upon withdrawal; broadly : persistent compulsive use of a substance known by the user to be*

harmful

Desire, in contrast, is defined as:

(A) conscious impulse toward something that promises enjoyment or satisfaction in its attainment.

The key difference between being addicted to pornography and simply desiring to view it, is the compulsion component in addiction. Those who are addicted to porn feel an irresistible impulse to use it. Using pornography becomes a habit, that when it's not present, there are physiological impacts – such as sexual dysfunction.

Sex is one of our most basic human needs. The drive to procreate is what ensures mankind survives. At our most base level, there are only three things that drive us:

- Nourishment
- Shelter, and
- Sex

Although watching pornography doesn't entirely fulfill the need to procreate, it can serve as a temporary replacement for many people. Additionally, for most, watching porn is physically exciting. There is something in Mankind's nature that enjoys watching others have sex.
However, we can also have a Pavlovian response to pornography. Sexual behaviors can quickly become reinforced using pornography. Think about it for a moment.

What's more physiologically rewarding than an orgasm?
Not much!

When you tie an activity, such as watching porn, to the reinforcement of having an orgasm, it shouldn't be surprising that your body would begin to crave pornography, tying the reward of orgasm to it. On top of this Pavlovian response, there's also a significant concern regarding desensitization of imagery.

Systematic desensitization is actually a therapy psychology professionals use to help patients overcome anxiety and phobias. This behavioral therapy typically begins with an image of what the patient is afraid of, slowly working them up to being able to remain calm when viewing the trigger for their phobia. Eventually, they become desensitized to the photo and move on to the actual item. The same desensitization can occur with pornographic images.

Pornography addiction can destroy a person's life. Marriages can be ruined. Jobs can be lost. Students can drop out of school. Although addiction is not the norm, most people who use pornography on an occasional basis don't become addicted, for some pornography addiction can be as devastating as an addiction to any illicit substance.

Possible signs of pornography addiction include:

- Continued porn use despite consequences and/or promises you've made to yourself or others to stop;
- Increasing amounts of time spent on pornography;
- Hours or even sometimes days spent viewing pornography;
- Viewing progressively more arousing, intense or bizarre sexual content;
- Lying, keeping secrets and covering up the nature or extent of porn use;
- Anger or irritability if asked to stop viewing porn;
- Reduced or even non-existent interest in sexual, physical and emotional connections with partners;
- Deeply rooted feelings of loneliness and detachment from other people;
- Drug or alcohol use or drug or alcohol addiction relapse connected with porn use;
- Increased objectification of strangers – seeing them as body parts rather than people;
- Escalation from viewing two-dimensional images to using the Internet to have anonymous sexual hook-ups or to find prostitutes.[1]

Pornography and Erectile Dysfunction

For men, one of the most significant concerns with the use of pornography is the potential for erectile dysfunction. This is a very real problem. According to Marnia Robinson of *Psychology Today*, porn-induced sexual dysfunction is a growing problem.[2]

In their recent article, they found that numerous men in their 20s who used Internet pornography were experiencing delayed ejaculation and sluggish erections when they were with real partners. In health forums across the web, men who admit to having a serious pornography/masturbation habit are having a hard time getting hard, with a real girl.

Robinson notes that there are threads concerning erectile dysfunction and pornography use springing up all over the Internet in a variety of forums, from bodybuilding to medical help to pick-up artists. Noticing this trend, *Psychology Today* began an ED and porn thread and with numerous respondents from different cultures, different education, different values, and different personalities, there was one commonality –

The use of Internet porn and the increasing need for more extreme material.

Many respondents saw their doctor and after a battery of tests were pronounced to be "just fine." In fact, many were told that their inability to perform with a partner was due to "performance anxiety."

Here's a simple test to tell if your erectile dysfunction with a partner truly is a performance anxiety issue:

- Masturbate alone, using only sensual touch - no porn and no fantasy.
- Use a similar speed and pressure as you would during sex.
- What's your erection quality like?

If you're not fully erect or if it takes a significant amount of effort to become erect, then chances are it's not performance anxiety.

Robinson notes more and more reports have come out connecting pornography addiction and sexual dysfunction. An Italian study, by Carlo Foresta, the head of the Italian Society of Andrology and Sexual Medicine and professor at the University of Padua, found that 70 percent of the men they were treating for sexual performance problems at their clinic had a heavy usage of Internet pornography. Other studies, such as Middlebury College's connecting erectile dysfunction to pornography, are showing very similar results – porn addiction can negatively affect your sexual performance!

Sadly, for many addicts who seek help with dysfunction, their healthcare professionals rarely discuss their use of pornography or masturbation, and their core problem remains untreated. To counter the effects of addiction, abstinence from porn and masturbation is typically the cure. Although many see improved performance after about 30 days of abstinence, neuroscience indicates that it can sometimes take more than a year for the pleasure pathways (those formed by the dopamine effect of orgasm) to return to normal. Counseling with a licensed therapist is also often required, to overcome true addiction, and couples therapy may be needed to help with relationship issues that have been a facet in the addiction.

Pornography and Penis Exercising – The Pros and Cons:

Using pornography with your penis exercising routine is fairly common, and can be quite effective. Oftentimes when performing exercises that require a constant erection for a long period of time, such as edging, jelqing or clamping, many guys think pornography can help keep their erection, while they think about the different aspect of the exercise – such as duration and quality. In today's busy world, porn can be a great tool to quickly get the erection needed to exercise effectively.

However, if the use of pornography goes beyond simply an exercising tool and becomes an engrained habit, there's the potential for addiction. It's a fine line that we have to walk when exercising, ensuring the use of porn doesn't become a compulsion that will then negatively affect us when we go to perform for our real life partners!

It all comes down to moderation. Using porn once in awhile to aid your penis exercises routine can help you get the enlargement results you want. However, in excess, you may get the enlargement results but then be unable to show off your growth when the time comes with your partner!

Part II Review

- ✓ Measuring is important as it allows you to track your progress, gain motivation with every inch you grow, and see if you are gaining.
- ✓ Always measure your erect length and girth the same way—this will allow you to consistently keep track of your growth.
- ✓ If you aim for nothing, you'll get nothing. Set a goal and you'll have a greater chance of getting the penis you want.
- ✓ Length is typically obtained through stretching exercises.
- ✓ Girth is typically obtained through expansion exercises.
- ✓ For the first week, give your penis at least two days of rest between workouts.
- ✓ In the beginning, less is more. Start out light and gradually increase the intensity overtime.
- ✓ Watch your body clues carefully. They are your flashlight on this journey.
- ✓ As with all exercising, side effects are possible.
- ✓ Pornography, in moderation, can be a useful addition for penis exercising.

The Fundamental Penis Exercises

Part III

In this part you will learn the fundamental exercises:

- The kegel
- The warm up
- The jelq
- The basic stretch

15

The Importance of the Kegel

"A hard man is good to find."

– *Mae West*

Over the years, several women—and even men—have told me that a hard penis is more important than a *big* one.

One woman I interviewed said, "The most important thing about a penis is its hardness. Who cares about penis size! Give me a penis that's rock-hard for a long period of time, and I'll keep coming back for more and more."

Another woman said, "A really hard penis is the biggest turn on of them all—simply because it shows that he really wants me."

It's true: a hard penis is the foundation of an optimal sex life. So it's surprising that there isn't more focus on penis hardness rather than penis size. But perhaps you're as hard as you want to be. Perhaps you always have the sexual stamina to please your partner the way she or he craves to be pleased. But maybe you don't. And if not, the kegel will help it happen. So, whether you're a soft man wanting to become hard, or a hard man wanting to become harder, the kegel is the number one exercise for the job. But the kegel doesn't stop there. Many men have experienced a long array of benefits from kegeling, such as:[1]

- Longer-lasting erections
- Multiple orgasms
- A cure for erectile dysfunction
- A cure for premature ejaculation
- A healthier prostate
- An improvement in penile blood flow
- An increase in intensity orgasm
- An increase in "shooting distance" when ejaculating
- An increase in control of ejaculation, which leads to greater sexual stamina
- An increase in angle of erection (for example, one man declared that his penis use to point towards the floor when erect, but now it points more straight out)
- An increase in penis size (generally caused by an improvement in blood flow)
- A cure for post-nucturition dribble (in which urine consistently dribbles from the penis at the end of an urination session)

Several penis exercisers have also reported that kegeling has helped enlarge the head of their penis. The head is considered one of the best parts of the penis to enlarge because it is the first part of your penis that your partner will feel during intercourse. So, to that end, the kegel is the first—and the most important—exercise you will learn. In fact, if you only do one exercise from this book, this is it.

The best part: the kegel is as simple as exercises come. It barely takes any time, and the multiple benefits makes the short time well spent. As far as penis exercises go, the kegel is also the only exercise that doesn't actually involve exercising your penis, but instead real skeletal muscles.

Look, No Hands!

The kegel strengthens your pelvic floor muscles, which are skeletal muscles in the same class as your biceps, triceps, and abs. The pelvic floor muscles are located at the "root" of the inner penis—roughly half of the penis is actually inside the body, and this half is encircled by the pelvic floor muscles (see Appendix B). The only way to exercise these muscles is with your mind, not with your hands. And because kegels require nothing but the will of your mind, you can kegel anywhere, anytime, without anyone ever knowing.

Healthy pelvic floor muscles are essential to a healthy penis. Many doctors and sexual experts define the pelvic floor muscles as the sex muscles because of their heavy influence on the penis and therefore sex. Strong pelvic floor muscles provide the benefits you just read previously, and weak pelvic floor muscles often result in weak erections and premature ejaculation.

Demoting the PC Muscle

Kegels were originally developed by gynecologist Arnold Kegel in the 1940s for women. Dr. Kegel observed that if women exercised their pubococcygeus (PC) muscle, then they would have a healthier pelvic region, a tighter vagina, and stronger orgasms. Some women even noticed an increase in sexual desire. Men later found that they too could reap sexual benefits by kegeling.

When men kegel they aren't exclusively using the PC muscle, which is well-established myth. A Registered Nurse and online moderator of Thunder's Place Penis Enlargement Forums named Steve "westla90069" Beal largely debunked this myth in is his essay Locating the BC Muscle. "Men and women are different," says Beal. "Females have essentially internal sex organs, males essentially external. The PC muscle is located in such a way that it is above and behind the penis and it contracts up into the pelvis. While its action on the rectum may add a little to the pull on the penis, it isn't the main muscle being exercised when men do kegels."

Men don't use just one sex muscle when they kegel—they use a whole set of muscles, largely the bulbocavernosus "BC" muscle and the ischiocavernosus "IC" muscle (see Appendix B for more on these muscles).[2] Kegeling makes both of these muscles stronger, which helps pump more blood into your penis. And as Dr. Steven Lamm, renowned author of The Hardness Factor, says, "Increasing blood flow to the penis strengthens erections and enhances the function of your vital organ."

Harder Than Viagra?

So how effective are kegels? A recent clinical study published in the *British Journal of General Practice* had 55 impotent men exercise their pelvic floor muscles with exercises like the kegel. Prior to the study, none of the men could maintain an erection for more than 30 seconds. By the study's end, 40 percent of the men had completely fixed their erectile dysfunction, and 35 percent of the men showed significant improvement.[3]

"The results were a real surprise . . . Strengthening up the pelvic floor muscles not only improved strength, but also endurance," said the lead scientist of the study, Dr. Grace Dorey, author of *Stronger and Longer* and visiting professor at the University of West England. "When men are going through a normal sex life, they should be looking to these exercises to extend their sex life. If men are performing reasonably well, this research would suggest that they may be able to improve their performance even further."

Dr. Frank Sommer, a German Urologist and professor at Hamburg University of Men's Health, conducted another study. The study involved 124 men who were separated into three groups. One group did pelvic floor exercises, one group took erection drugs (such as Viagra), and one group took a placebo (such as a salt pill). The pelvic exercise group took the lead with 80 percent experiencing stronger and harder erections, followed by the erection drug group with 74 percent, and the placebo group with 18 percent.

Kegels Help the Prostate

In The Prostate Health Program, authors Daniel W. Nixon, M.D., and Max Gomez, Ph.D., point out that exercising the pelvic floor muscles amplifies the circulation and stimulation of the prostate.

"When performed properly, Kegel exercises force blood into your penis and genital area, benefiting both the prostate and the urinary tract. In addition, Kegel exercises indirectly massage the prostate," says Gomez and Nixon.

"Kegel exercises are also great for improving virility (potency) and achieving greater ejaculation and arousal control," Gomez and Nixon affirm. "This impacts very favorably on the prostate, since a healthy sex life often equals a healthy prostate."

A healthy prostate is important because behind lung cancer, prostate cancer is the second most common cancer in men. Approximately one out of ten men will be diagnosed with the disease. And here's the really bad news: the majority of men will have a problem with their prostate before they die. Whether it's prostate cancer, prostate enlargement or prostate infection, each can have an ill effect on your penis, your sex, and ultimately your life.

16

Kegel Exercises

All this talk of pelvic floor muscles might have your head spinning more than The Beatles' All You Need is Love disc in the late 60s. But kegeling is about as easy as it gets. The hardest part is locating the right muscles. But as long as you have a place to use the bathroom, whether it is the urinal at work, your backyard, or even your ex-girlfriend's kitchen sink, you'll be counting kegels in no time.

Finding Your Pelvic Floor Muscles

1. Go to the restroom and urinate.
2. Stop urinating mid-flow. The muscles used to clamp off your urine are your pelvic floor muscles. You should feel the muscles contract every time you stop urinating. If you didn't feel it, try stopping again. This time, place two fingers on your perineum—the area between your testicles and anus—while stopping. You should be able to feel your muscles contracting with your fingers.
3. Once you locate the muscles, contract them when you aren't urinating. *Each contraction is a kegel.*

Kegel Exercise 1: The Kegel Start/Stop

The method used to find your pelvic floor muscles, stopping your urine mid-flow, is actually an exercise in itself. From this point on, every time you go to the restroom, stop mid-flow for several seconds, and then restart. Do this at least three times. Don't be shy though; if you have the time (and the urine) to start/stop six, seven, and even eight times in one session, go for it. This exercise is not only useful for building stronger pelvic floor muscles, but it's also useful for continually reminding yourself where your pelvic floor muscles are.

The kegel start/stop is the *only* exercise in this book that you should do every single day, as it's rarely ever intense enough to cause over-training Doing this exercise every day has similar improvements on your penis health as walking every day does on your physical health.

Exercising Your Pelvic Floor Muscles

Along with doing the kegel start/stop every time you use the restroom, you will exclusively exercise your pelvic floor muscles three to four times a week. In the beginning, try to get at least one day of rest between each kegel workout. Similar to your other muscles, your pelvic floor muscles become stronger during rest, not during exercise.

During your first week, you will spend only one minute on kegels per each workout. As the weeks goes on, you will increase this to five minutes or more. It won't be hard to find a few minutes of time, as it's easy to multitask while kegeling. You can kegel while watching television, while driving, while washing dishes, while browsing the web, and even while you're at work. Anywhere, anytime. Sitting in a dull

Kill Driving Time

Several men Kegel while driving. One penis exerciser timed his kegels with the stop lights: he would Kegel when the light turned green, and hold the contraction until he hit the next red light.

meeting? Go for it. No one will ever know.

The next two exercises are good for kegel beginners. After the first five weeks, you can add advanced kegel exercises (found in Appendix C).

Kegel Exercise 2: The Kegel

This exercise is a simple contraction of your pelvic floor muscles. You can do this exercise fully clothed or naked.

The exercise:

Contract your pelvic floor muscles for one to two seconds, then release. Each contraction is one kegel repetition.

It's That Easy!

Doing just one minute of regular kegels and the kegel start/stop every time you use the restroom is often all it takes to dramatically boost your hardness and penis health.

Kegel Exercise 3: The Kegel Slam

Whenever you're ready, try this next exercise, the kegel slam. Men with strong pelvic floor muscles will be able to do this exercise within a few days of doing regular kegels. Men with weak pelvic floor muscles will need a month or more of strengthening the muscles for this exercise.

The exercise:

Over five seconds time, slowly contract your pelvic floor muscles as tight as possible. Subsequently hold the tight contraction for another five seconds. Then take another five seconds to slowly release the contraction. All three steps (the slow contraction, the hold, and the release) should take roughly fifteen seconds to complete.

Kegel Assignment

- Locate your pelvic floor muscles by stopping your urine mid-flow.
- From this point on, do the kegel start/stop at least three times *every time* you use the restroom.
- Do 3 sets of 20 kegels (for a total of 60 kegels). This is equivalent to roughly 1 to 2 minutes of kegeling. If you find it easier, break this up throughout the day. For example, you can do twenty kegels in the morning, twenty in the afternoon, and twenty in the evening.

Reverse Kegels

As the name implies, a reverse kegel is the opposite of a kegel. The goal is to stretch the pelvic floor muscles, pushing down on the PC and BC muscles. Reverse kegels are an important part of ensuring you have a balanced pelvic floor. Performing kegels can often result in overtraining. With a balanced pelvic floor, you will have better control of your erections, and a reverse kegel can be performed during sex to bring you back from the PONR. Learn more about reverse kegels and prevention of premature ejaculation, on page 198.

As with performing a kegel, the first step is to recognize your pelvic floor muscles. One of the easiest ways to accomplish this is by stopping your urine midstream. Those are your PC and BC muscles you're using to stop the urine. For the reverse kegel, however, the movement you want is the relaxing of this muscle when you let the urine flow. It is a pushing down of the pelvic floor some compare to the motion of farting.

Perform a daily routine of both repetitive short pushes of the muscles and holding the push for up to 30 seconds. Be sure to exhale while performing the reverse kegel, to create a force against your push. Like kegels, reverse kegels can be performed any time of day, anywhere. Performing light reverse kegels throughout your day will help restore your pelvic floor balance.

17

Kegel Pitfalls

When learning how to kegel, you may find yourself falling through a few common trap doors.

Pitfall 1: Improperly Kegeling

In *Dr. Peter Scardino's Prostate Book*, Scardino says one in four to five men do kegel exercises improperly; and when they are done improperly, they aren't effective. "It is important that your stomach, upper thighs, and buttocks, are all completely relaxed when kegeling. They should not be moving," says Dr. Barbara Keesling in *How to Make Love All Night*.

For this reason, you'll want to learn how to kegel while you're sitting down. Moving and using your other muscles, especially your legs, makes it hard to isolate and strengthen your pelvic floor muscles. Also, for the first few days, place two fingers on your perineum while you kegel. Touching your perineum while kegeling will allow you to feel your pelvic floor muscles in action and recognize when you are doing the kegel effectively.

If after a week you are still unable to isolate your pelvic floor muscles effectively, try doing what Dr. Keesling suggests: "exhaust the other muscles first so they don't interfere with your new exercise regimen." For example, if you're constantly tensing your abs while kegeling, do a few sit ups beforehand.

Pitfall 2: Over-training

Like any other exercise, over-training applies to the kegel too. In fact, you'll want take extra precaution in gradually working your way up with kegels, as you're exercising skeletal muscles. Over-trained pelvic floor muscles can lead to temporary erectile dysfunction and temporary premature ejaculation—neither of which is fun. So start out light and get adequate rest. As time goes on, you can eventually move up to kegeling five or more minutes a day.

> **HIS STORY**
> **Too Much Kegeling**
>
> Here's what one man said about his initial problems with kegeling: "I use to kegel 20 minutes a day, every day. I did this for at least three months and finally gave up when I didn't notice any difference. I kept thinking that these guys are nuts; this kegel stuff doesn't work! Finally, a few months ago, I learned that it's best to give my "kegel muscles" a break every day or so. Ever since, I've been kegeling only three times a week (Sunday, Tuesday, and Friday) with great results. Now I know that these muscles are like your biceps—they need rest!"

Pitfall 3: Too Much Sensitivity

The kegel is famous for increasing penile sensitivity, which is great for sexual pleasure. The increased sensitivity, however, occasionally causes a temporary side effect: It's too sensitive for some men and this can lead to temporary premature ejaculation. If this occurs, your penis should adapt to the sensitivity within a few weeks.

If you are unconsciously kegeling during sex, premature ejaculation can also occur.

18

The Importance of Warming Up

While the kegel is an exercise that can be done anywhere, the other penis exercises usually need to be done in a sit-down workout session. Also unlike kegels, the other penis exercises require you to warm up first. If you have ever actively exercised, you were most likely taught the significance of warming up. Although the warm up is much different when performing penis exercises, the concept is still the same. Warming up before performing penis exercises increases growth and decrease chances of injury.

A warm up, which literally involves heating the penis, is often more important than the actual exercises. A warm up helps you avoid several of the unwanted side effects, such as red spots and the darkening effect. Just as important, a bad warm up or no warm up at all can stop you from gaining.

The Importance of Heat

Temperature has a significant effect on your penis. "During moments of anxiety or when a man is cold, the penis shrinks up. When feeling comfortable or warm, the penis will fill up like a water balloon, even without sexual arousal," says Abraham Morgentaler, associate

Clinical Professor at Harvard Medical School and author of *Male Body*.

You most likely already know how temperature can influence your penis size, shape and feeling. If you've ever been swimming in a cold pool, you probably experienced the turtle effect—in which your penis became stiff and shrank like a turtle's head into its shell. The turtle effect occurs because your body is keeping warm your important organs, such as your heart and lungs, while decreasing blood flow to your not-so important organ, the penis (yes, your penis might be your favorite organ, but it's not essential to you living). Heat has the opposite effect of cold: it increases blood flow to your penis along with making it more flexible and easier to stretch.

Heat = Flexible Tissue

Heat makes the penis more flexible, more relaxed, and less stiff. The main reason for warming up is so when you're exercising you aren't tearing stiff tissues within your penis. Instead, you're exercising relaxed, flexible tissue. It's easy to see how increased flexibility can lead to more gains. The more flexible your penis, the easier it stretches, and the more it enlarges.

Heat = Increased Blood Flow

Heat also acts upon your arteries like Drano does your kitchen pipes—it opens them up. As a result, a warm up increases blood flow to your penis. With more blood flowing to your penis, your erections will be harder, healthier and your workouts more effective.

Always Warm Up

For one reason or another, many men skip out on the warm up. This is not advised. A warm up is essential to healthy and effective penis exercises. Every time a man asks me if it's okay to skip warming up, I come back with the same answer: If you are exercising your penis to make it bigger and harder, then why skip something that will ultimately maximize growth and minimize injury.

19

Warming Up, It's That Easy

A warm up involves applying heat to your penis for five to ten minutes prior to performing penis exercises. As you can imagine, heat can be applied through a variety of ways. Moist heat and infrared (IR) heat are the most effective. The three most popular warm ups that provide moist heat are: a moist heating pad, a rice sock, and a warm wash cloth. Infrared heat can be applied with an IR lamp or an IR massager. Let's go over these warm ups in more detail, and then you'll learn how to warm up.

Moist Heating Pad

Moist heating pads are generally used to relieve pain and muscle spasms. They usually plug into an outlet and take a few minutes to reach desired temperature. Moist heating pads are fairly cheap and are sold at nearly any retail store.

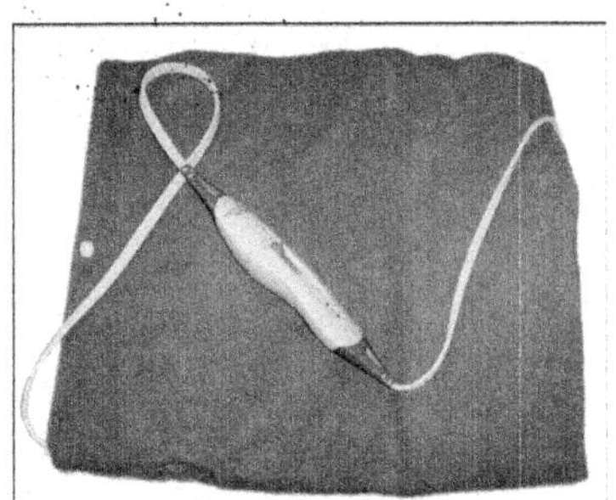

Moist Heating Pad

Rice Sock

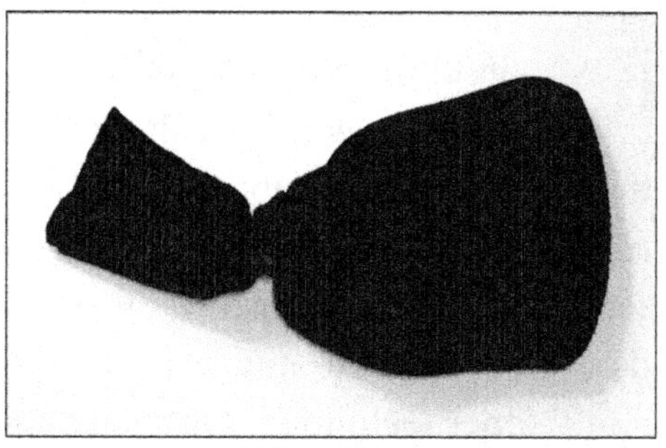

Rice Sock

A rice sock is convenient and inexpensive—it's made with three items sitting around your house. To make a *rice sock* you need:

1. A sock—any sock that fits around your penis will do, but cotton socks tend to work best.
2. Uncooked rice—it doesn't matter if it's white, wheat, or wild, as long as it's uncooked.
3. A microwave.

Once you have the above materials, prepare a rice sock by following these three steps:

1. Take your sock and fill it with approximately one to two cups of uncooked rice.
2. Tie the sock shut. Make sure to leave enough room in the sock so you can comfortably move it around your penis.
3. Put the rice sock in the microwave and heat for approximately 30 to 90 seconds or until you reach desired temperature.

Tip!

Put a cup of water into the microwave with the rice sock. The steam from the hot water will help to humidify the rice, thus making the sock even more effective when applied to your penis.

Warm Wash Cloth

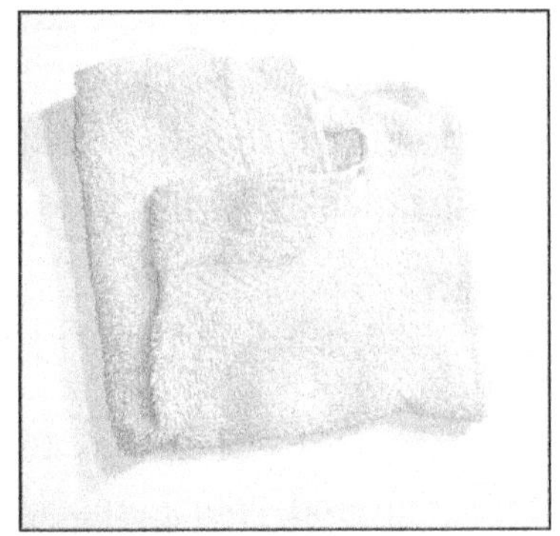

Warm Wash Cloth

Although a warm wash cloth is one of the simplest warm up aids—all you do is run it under hot water—it's the least effective. That's because a wash cloth tends to cool down much more quickly than any other technique. Only use a warm wash cloth when the other options are out of the question.

Infrared Massager

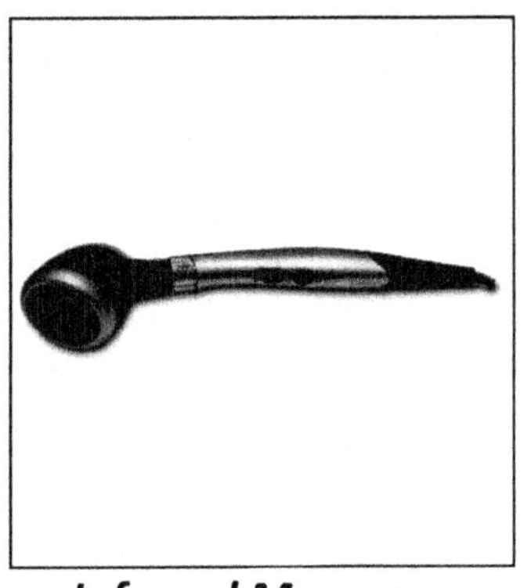

Infrared Massager

Infrared heat is able to warm up the penis best as it heats the deeper tissues in the penis, says Richard Howard II, Dr. PH, an experienced penis exerciser who has gained over three inches in length and two inches in girth. An IR massager is also great because massage increases circulation, improves blood flow, and—as anybody who has had a massage will attest—relaxes tissue. Combine these effects with the benefits that an IR warm up already provides, and you have a penis that is exceedingly flexible and ready to expand.

Another good warm up that produces infrared heat is an IR heat lamp. Although it doesn't have the massage factor, it does allow you to keep heat on your penis during the entire workout. With a lamp, though, you'll want to be extra careful not to burn yourself. As with all lamps, you must keep it a safe distance from your body – at least 18 inches from your penis and anywhere from 24 to 36 inches is even better. Dr. Howard recommends that you keep the lamp a safe distance, follow the instructions, avoid using too many watts, and use your intuition. If you follow these precautions and use prudence, it's as safe as any other heating device.

Infrared massagers are sold at most retail stores and at wellness stores. Infrared heat lamps can be found at most pet stores in the reptile section. You can also find an IR bulb at most retails stores if you already have a lamp.

Other Warm Ups

A few other common ways to warm up include:

- Using a steamed towel
- Using a moist heating pack
- Using a heated gel pack
- Placing your penis into a thermal mug with hot water
- Sitting in a sauna or spa
- Standing in a hot shower or sitting in a hot bath

Warming Up: Step-by-Step

Once you have chosen your warm up method, follow the steps below prior to every penis exercises workout:

1. Prepare the warm up. If you are using a heating pad or an IR massager, plug it in and let it heat up. If you are using a rice sock, warm it up in the microwave. If you are using a wash cloth, run it under hot water.
2. Once you've reached the desired temperature, check the warm up with your hand. If it's too hot, let it cool down to a comfort level. A good rule of thumb: lukewarm isn't hot enough and burning is too hot.
3. Once the warm up material is heated, cover your entire penis and keep it wrapped for ten minutes. If you are using a rice sock, wrap it around your penis—don't put it in the sock with the rice. If you are using an IR massager, move it around and massage the entire penis. If the warm up gets cold, then reheat and reapply.
4. As soon as you've warmed up, start performing penis exercises.

Extra Warm Up Tips!

Avoid the family jewels:

Heat kills sperm count. Try covering your testicles with a thick sock, or putting on a pair of thick underwear and bringing your penis through the pee-hole. Covering your testicles is especially important if you use infrared heat to warm up your penis, as it penetrates tissues deepest. So if you warm up with IR heat, always do a double take to make sure the little guys are covered up. This goes double time if you're trying to conceive.

Start exercising immediately after you warm up:

Do this or else the heat will quickly dissipate. Also, the sooner you start exercising, the more flexible your penis will be.

Use heat during your penile workout:

This can be done in a variety of ways, such as doing your penis exercises in the shower, bath, sauna, or hot tub. Many penis exercisers also place a rice sock on their penis while stretching or focus on IR light on their penis while exercising.

Try gently massaging your penis while warming up:

Even if you don't use an IR massager to warm up, give your penis a quick massage pre-workout. Depending on what kind of warm up you are using, you may even be able to directly massage your penis with the actual warm up material. Steamed towels, for example, work well for massaging the penis. If you warm up in the shower, use your hands to massage your penis.

Warm up your perineum (the area between your testicles and anus):

Your inner penis (the part of the penis that's inside your body) is located beneath the perineum. Warming up this area makes your inner penis easier to stretch, and thus easier to bring outside of your body. You should also warm up the area near your pubic bone, as this will make your ligaments stretch more easily. For a better understanding of your perineum, inner penis, and ligaments see Appendix B: The Penis Anatomy.

Thoroughly warm up:

Heat every aspect of your penis thoroughly, or else you will be doing little more than heating your skin. Apply heat to the base, the top, the bottom, and the sides of your penis (again, avoid heating your testicles). If you do your warm up in the shower, position yourself so that the hot water is hitting your entire penis.

Warm Up Assignment

Your homework is to make a choice. Choose your warm up. The type of warm up you choose is a matter of preference and convenience.

20

On the Safe Side

"See, the problem is that God gave men a brain and a penis, but only enough blood to run one at a time."

– Robin Williams

As you embark on the next two exercises—the jelq and the basic stretch—you will actually mold, build, and exercise your penis. These two exercises will lay the groundwork for every other penis exercise you will learn. Before you learn these exercises, you'll want to take a few precautions to keep your penile workouts healthy and injury-free. In addition to warming up, use the following guidelines:

Never grip, pull on, or stroke the head of your penis:

The head is the most delicate and sensitive part of your penis, so treat it well.

Let it rest:

Not only should you give your penis time to rest between workout days, but also between exercises. Every few minutes, give your penis a few seconds break.

Avoid doing exercises erect, especially in the beginning:

Do not jelq or stretch erect.

Take your time:

This can't be stressed enough. The biggest mistake beginner's make is rushing through the whole process in an effort to speed things up. This almost never works and often leads to over-training and softer erections.

While learning these next two exercises, it is recommended you make it your priority to practice getting your technique down and becoming familiar with the idea of exercising your penis. Each exercise has illustrated pictures and instructions. Read the steps thoroughly to make sure you are performing each exercise properly. For your convenience, you can also find videos of the exercises on the online companion to this book, http://www.PEGym.com/penis-exercises.

21

Jelqing

The jelq is the foundation of penis exercises. No matter what you're exercising your penis for—to gain girth, length, or hardness—the jelq will help you get there. The jelq works so well because it uses an OK-grip to push your blood, and the nutrients within it, throughout your penis. The jelq also builds pressure within the penis' smooth muscle, blood vessels, and other tissues. Overtime, the stress of this pressure causes the penis to expand, enlarge, and harden—similar to how putting stress on your muscles causes them to become stronger and harder.

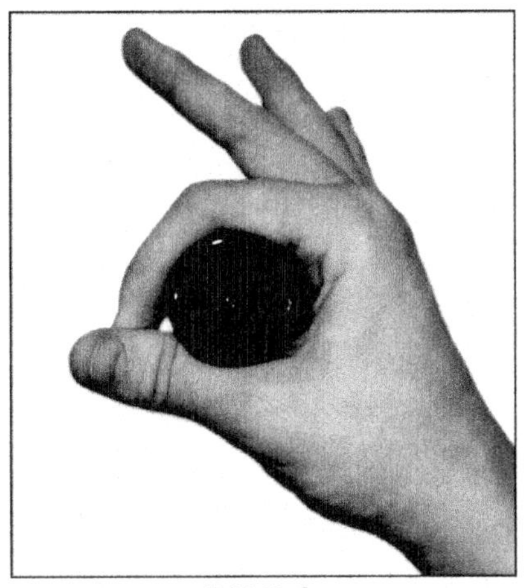

OK Grip

A common question is, "Where did the jelq come from?" Oddly enough, the jelq's origin is largely a mystery. Some sources speculate it has been around for roughly 30 years, and is nothing more than a fine art of masturbating; others suggest that the jelq is an ancient Arabic exercise. Regardless of the jelq's origins, its popularity is wide-spread on the Internet and in the penis enlargement community. And for good reason—many men have gained inches from just this one exercise.

Lubrication Required

To jelq you'll need a lubricant, such as baby oil. Eventually, you may be able to get by without using lubrication, but stick with it for now. Lubrication is gentle on the skin, which helps you overcome some of the unwanted side effects such as skin darkening. It also makes the learning process easier.

Good Lubricants

The best lubricants don't have to be continually reapplied. Below is a list of popular lubricants that have worked for many penis exercisers.

- Baby oil (the best baby oil has added vitamin E and aloe, as both are healthy for the skin)
- Canola oil
- Vegetable oil
- Olive oil
- Coconut oil
- Cocoa butter
- K-Y jelly
- Astroglide
- Vaseline
- Essential Vein Oil
- Penis exercising oils

Essential Vein Oil

Essential Vein Oil (EVO) was made for the sole purpose of performing penis exercises. For that reason, EVO is a more beneficial lubricant, but it's also more expensive. Created by a penis exerciser who uses the online alias Eroset, EVO combines several essential oils and herbs that are vasodilators — meaning they open your blood vessels and increase blood flow. As a result, EVO is great for increasing hardness and overall penile health. The downfall of EVO is that you have to make it yourself. For a list of ingredients and instructions on how to make EVO, see Appendix D: Penis Exercising Resources.

Penis Exercising Oils

If you don't want to make your own lubricant, such as EVO, but want to find a lubricant with vasodilators and other ingredients specific to improving penile hardness, go to http://www.PEGym.com/penis-lubricants. There you can find user reviews of all the popular lubricants.

Bad Lubricants

The worst lubricants are water, lotions, and soaps. Water is a bad lubricant because it doesn't last for more than a few jelq strokes. Lotions and soaps are bad because they often cause skin irritation and make your penis itch.

22

Your Erection Level

When you jelq, you'll need to consider your erection level—how engorged your penis is. You don't want to jelq too erect because it can be potentially dangerous. On the other hand, you don't want to jelq without any engorgement or the jelq won't be effective.

To help you decipher how erect your penis should be when jelqing and doing other exercises, this chapter has a detailed description of the five different erection levels. Each erection level is gauged by percentage. A full-blown erection is a 100 percent erection level. An absolutely flaccid penis is a 0 percent erection level. Use the following "erection gauge" to help you with all the penis exercises throughout the book.

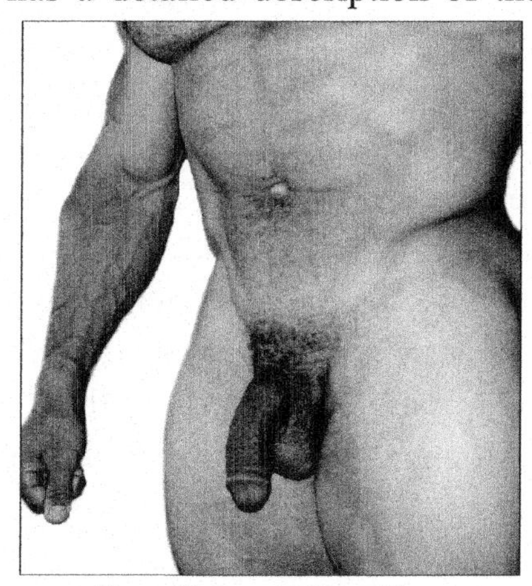

Zero Percent Erection

Zero Percent Erection Level

The penis is in a completely flaccid state. With a zero percent

percent erection level, the penis is in its smallest and least erect state. With some men, their flaccid penis is always at a zero percent erection level. Other men only experience a zero percent erection level on rare occasions —when they swim in a cold pool, for example.

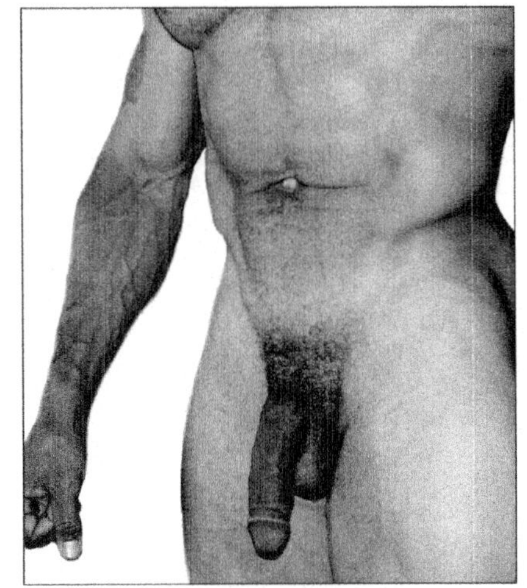
25 Percent Erection

25 Percent Erection Level

The penis is in a flaccid state. With a 25 percent erection level, the penis is flaccid; but it is filled with more blood and often feels more flexible than a 0 percent erection level. Most stretches are done with a 25 percent erection level.

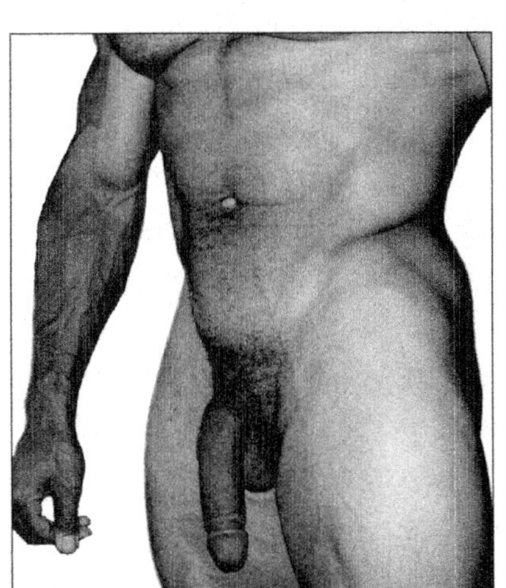
50 Percent Erection

50 Percent Erection Level

The penis is in a fully-pumped flaccid state. With a 50 percent erection level, the penis is still flaccid; but it is pumped with blood and much larger than a 0 percent erection level. A penis with a 50 percent erection level is near the size of the erect penis, but with no firmness or hardness whatsoever. In this state, the penis can be moved, bent, and squeezed without any resistance. Some girth exercises are performed with a 50 percent erection level.

75 Percent Erection Level

The penis is in a semi-erect state. With a 75 percent erection level, the penis is nearly full of blood. In this state, the penis still can be moved, bended, jelqed, and squeezed; but with slight resistance. A semi-erect penis has minor firmness and hardness, but generally isn't hard enough to penetrate the vagina for sex. Various girth exercises are performed in this erection level.

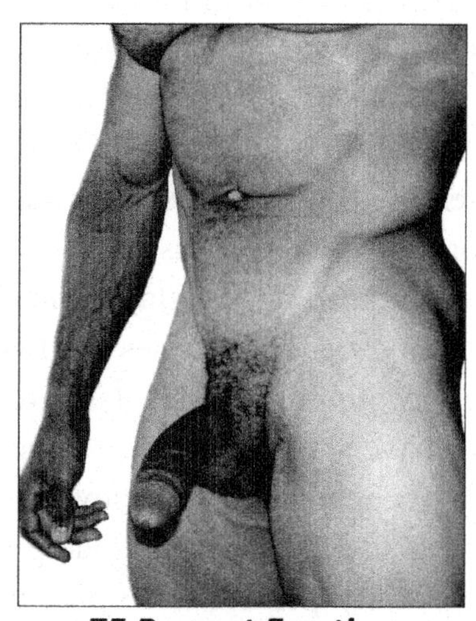

75 Percent Erection

100 Percent Erection Level

The penis is in a completely erect state. With a 100 percent erection level, the penis is full of blood and can penetrate a vagina with ease. In this state, the penis provides great resistance and is much harder to move, bend, jelq, and squeeze. Avoid exercising in this state until you have been exercising for at least three months—and possibly much longer. Penis exercising with a 100 percent erection level is dangerous if your penis isn't conditioned to the exercises. And even if it is conditioned, for the most part you'll want to avoid exercising your penis with an erection.

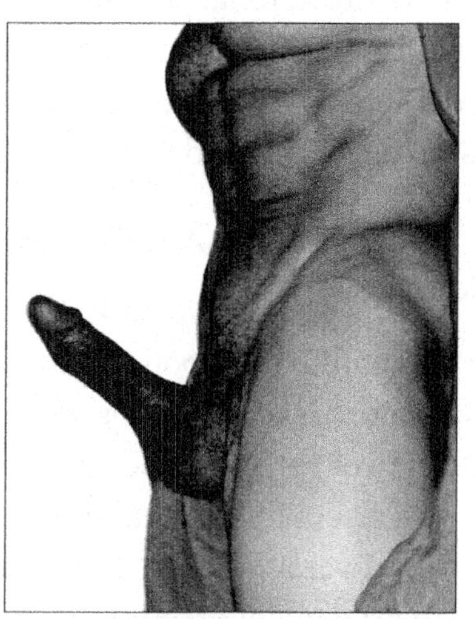

100 Percent Erection

Jelqing With a Proper Erection Level

As a general rule: The higher your erection level, the less flexible your penis, and the more intense the exercise. In the beginning, you'll want to jelq with an erection level between 40 and 75 percent. Jelqing with less than 40 or 50 percent is unproductive because it doesn't efficiently push blood throughout your penis. Jelqing with more than 75 percent is dangerous when you first start out because your penis isn't conditioned for performing penis exercises.

To keep it safe, stay in the 40 to 75 percent range until you've been performing penis exercises for two months. After that, you can gradually increase your erection level and thus the amount of intensity. In the future, you'll have the opportunity to perform some jelq-like advance exercises with a 95 percent erection level, but even with these exercises you should still be able to move the blood up your penis without having to force it.

Many penis exercisers find that jelqing at higher erection levels obtains more girth, whereas jelqing at lower erection levels obtains more length. Try different variations to see what works best for you. But never jelq with a 100 percent erection level. Your penis is resistant to change when it's erect, and forcing anything on your erect penis is like forcing pressure on an inflated tire.

Are You a Grower or a Shower?

A grower typically has a small flaccid penis that grows exceptionally upon erection. The average flaccid size of a grower is usually around a 0 to 25 percent erection level. A shower (pronounced *sh oh 'er*) is good for "show" and has a big flaccid penis that doesn't enlarge that much upon erection. The average flaccid size of a shower is generally around a 50 to 60 percent erection level. According to an international Men's Health survey, 79 percent of men are growers and 21 percent of men are showers.

23

Jelqing: Step-by-Step

Jelqing doesn't require extreme pressure for it to work. The goal is to push the blood up the penis, not force it. Use a graceful, light grip.

Starting Position

You can either sit or stand while doing this exercise, but many men find that it's most comfortable to sit down with their legs spread apart. Either way, keep your back straight and allow gravity to do its work—centralizing the blood to your pelvic region.

Erection Level

Your erection level should be between 40 and 75 percent.

> *Remember* to warm up for ten minutes before attempting the jelq.

The Jelq

1. Lather your penis with lubrication and bring your penis to desired erection level.

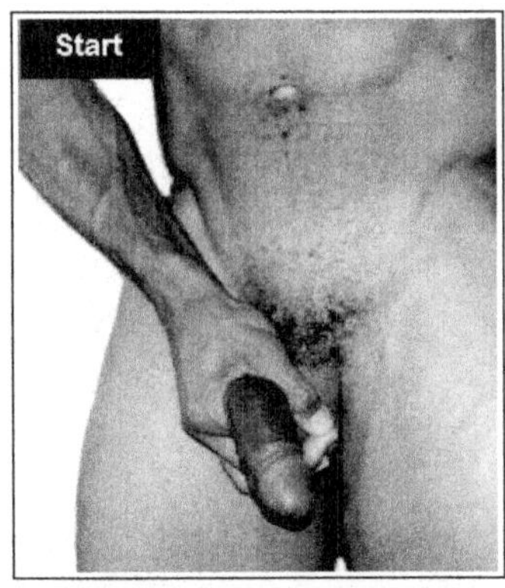

2. With either hand, use your thumb and pointer finger to create an OK-grip around the base of your penis. Place the grip as close to the pubic bone as possible.

3. Apply pressure to the grip and slowly move it up the penis. The ideal pressure is one that does not hurt, but effectively milks your penis.

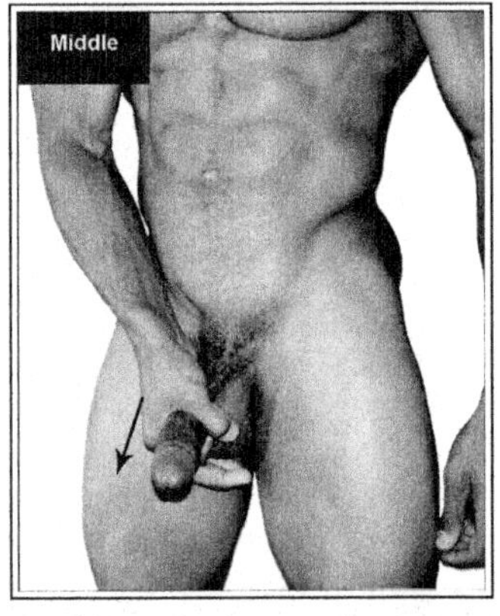

4. Stop the grip directly before you reach the head (do not jelq the head of your penis). You have completed one jelq. Each jelq should take approximately two to three seconds.

5. Immediately take your other hand and repeat the same process. Switch hands each rep until you reach the desired number of reps.

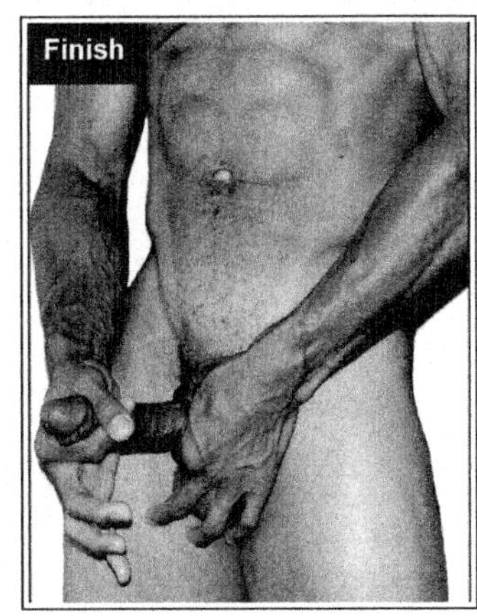

Extra Jelq Tips!

Add a stretch:

If part of your goal is to gain length, then give your penis a quick tug after each jelq. This light, gentle stretch should take no more than half a second.

Jelq backwards:

Several penis exercisers attest that jelqing in a backwards motion has allowed them to build a thicker base. To jelq backwards, simply push the blood towards the base of your penis rather than towards the head.

Use time as your counter:

You can record your workouts two ways. The first way is to count reps. Counting reps can become tiresome when you are doing an exercise that requires more than a hundred reps. The second way is to use time as your counter. For example, a jelq lasts roughly two to three seconds, which translates into roughly 250 jelqs every ten minutes. Many men find that timing ten minutes is easier than counting all 250 jelqs.

If you're uncircumcised, try pulling back your foreskin:

It doesn't matter if you're uncircumcised or circumcised when performing penis exercises. However, many uncircumcised men report that it's more comfortable to use one hand to draw back the foreskin and the other hand to jelq.

Avoid placing pressure on the top of your penis:

Your dorsal nerve runs along the top of your penis and it is like the spinal cord of your penis sensitivity. In short, it allows your penis to keenly feel sensation. If you place an exorbitant amount of pressure on this sensitive area, you may cause damage that could temporarily lead to less sensitivity.

Common Jelqing Questions!

"Is there another way to grip when jelqing?"

The OK-grip is the most common grip, but it's not the only one. Anything that pushes blood up your penis will work. Another notable grip is the pincher grip. To form the pincher grip, place your index finger on one side of your penis and your thumb on the other side. When complete, the grip looks as if you are pinching your penis.

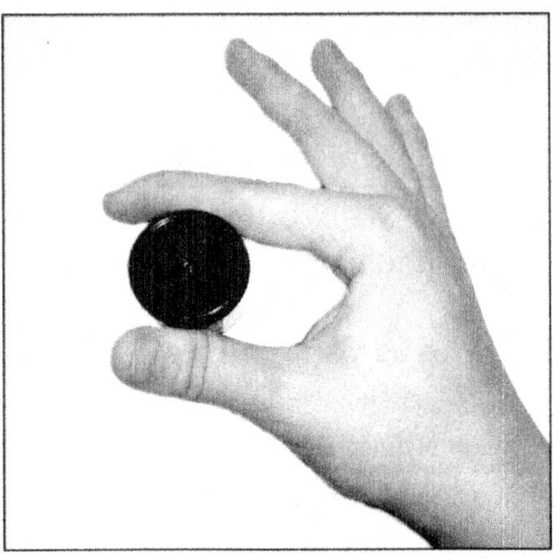

Pincher Grip

Both the OK-grip and pincher grip are effective. The pincher grip, however, puts less pressure on both the underside and the head of your penis. For variety, switch it up and rotate the two grips. For another variation of the pincher grip, put your index finger on the underside of your penis and your thumb on the upper side.

"Do I really need a lubricant to jelq?"

Not exactly, but I recommend that you use lubrication to learn how to jelq. Think of it this way: Lubrication is to jelqing as training wheels are to riding a bicycle. Jelqing without lubrication—also known as dry jelqing—causes skin irritation for several men, which often leads to darkening of the penis and other unwanted side effects. Skin irritation is especially more apt to occur in the beginning, when you are first learning how to jelq.

Yet, after the initial two or three weeks, many men find that the skin irritation is minimal. So once you master the jelq, feel free to experiment. The dry jelq may not cause you any problems. If you attempt dry jelqing, use a lighter grip than when wet jelqing.

Another way you can dry jelq—and possibly avoid skin irritation —is to keep the OK-grip in constant contact with the same spot of skin for the entire jelq (rather than pushing the grip up the skin). Using this method, it may be hard to complete a jelq with one single stroke (from the base to the head). Therefore, jelqing the shaft in two or three strokes might be necessary. For example, start at the base of your penis and jelq to mid-shaft Then re-grip and go from mid-shaft to the head of your penis. (Note: many men have trouble understanding this exercise with words and pictures alone. For more clarity, go to http://www.pegym.com for a video.)

If you find that the skin irritation isn't a problem for you, dry jelqing does have its pros. The biggest pro of dry jelqing is that it's great if you're performing penis exercises in secrecy and you are not telling your significant other, as it doesn't require cleaning up lubrication afterward. Dry jelqing is also easy to do in places where wet jelqing is impracticable. For example, you can perform a few dry jelqs during bathroom breaks. Another pro of dry jelqing is that it's less arousing, which is beneficial if you find yourself continually getting erect while jelqing.

Another alternative that doesn't require lubrication is using a jelq simulator. This device provides the same effect as the jelq, often with even more consistency, and generally doesn't require the use of a lubricant. You can read more about jelq simulators in Appendix A under the section "Penis Enlargement Devices."

"I always get an erection when I try to jelq. How do I fix it?"

The jelq is an arousing exercise. Eventually, with enough practice, you will be able to rise above this problem. In the meantime:

- Try to calm your arousal with your mind. Take deep breaths and relax.
- Stop, let your erection subside, and resume.

- Use the pincher grip to focus the pressure on the left and right side of your penis. Switching to the pincher grip often works because the OK-grip stimulates the underside of your penis, which is an extremely arousing area.
- Try getting up and walking around for a minute or two while you jelq. This will circulate your blood throughout your body.
- If all else fails, try dry jelqing.

Jelq Assignment

1. Obtain a lubricant
2. Jelq for ten minutes (approximately 250 jelqs)

24

Stretching

While the jelq works by forcing blood all throughout the penis, the stretch is much more basic. As you can imagine, stretching is a simple process. Compare penile stretching to stretching a rubber band. When you stretch a rubber band for the first few times, it typically goes back to its normal size. But if you stretch the same rubber band over and over, it will eventually become longer. Similarly, a single penile stretch doesn't cause growth. Instead, penis growth occurs through multiple stretches over time.

Stretching is possibly the oldest form of penis exercises and is indispensable to any man trying to gain length. It also increases hardness, so you'll want to do at least four or five minutes of stretching even if your main goal isn't more length.

Not Tug Of War

The goal of stretching is to slowly accustom your penis to the stress. Key word: slowly. Your penis doesn't react well to sudden, quick stretches. The more sudden the stretch, the more likely you'll injure your penis, and the less likely you'll gain. So avoid pulling as if you're in a tug of war contest, especially in the beginning. At first, start with slow and gentle stretches.

25

Basic Stretching: Step-by-Step

The basic stretch is the backbone of all length exercises. Once you get the hang of this exercise, the other stretches will come naturally.

Starting Position

You can stretch while standing, sitting, or laying down.

Erection Level

Your erection level should be between 0 and 40 percent. In the beginning, avoid stretching with an erection level much more than your typical flaccid penis.

> *Remember* to warm up for ten minutes. If you just warmed up so you could jelq, then you do not have to warm up again.

The Basic Stretch:

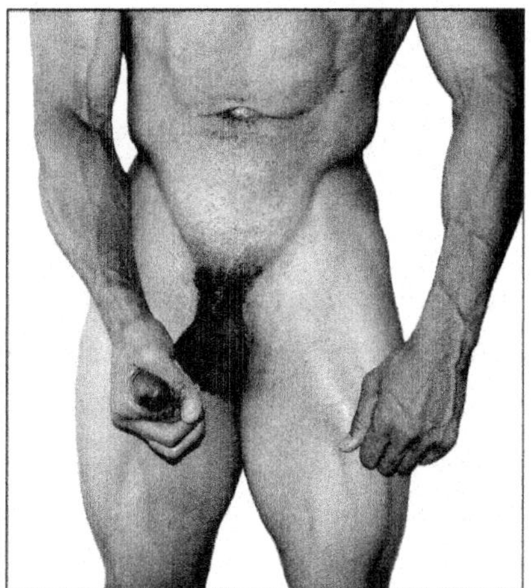

1. Grip your penis. Anywhere will do, so long as you don't directly grip the head.
2. Gently pull **straight out** for 30 seconds.
3. After the stretch, quickly restore blood circulation by either kegeling or gently slapping your penis against your leg.
4. Repeat steps 1 through 3, but stretch your penis in the following directions for 30 seconds each:
   - **Down**, penis pointing towards the floor
   - **Up**, penis pointing towards the ceiling
   - **Right**, penis pointing to the right
   - **Left**, penis pointing to the left

Common Stretching Questions!

"Will I lose girth by stretching?"

No, stretching generally doesn't cause a loss in girth. In fact, when combined with the jelq and girth exercises (which you'll use after you advance), stretching may actually help increase girth. That's because after stretching, the tissues within the penis are already flexible and submissive. Combine the increase flexibility with girth exercises or jelqing, then the penis will continue to stretch, but in an outward direction. Several penis exercisers also report an increase in girth at their base—near the pubic bone—because of stretching.

"Can I hold the stretch longer than 30 seconds?"

When you first start out, keep your stretches to a maximum hold of thirty seconds each. Over the next five weeks, work your way up to sixty to ninety second holds.

"What should I feel when stretching?"

Many men feel different things when they stretch. Several penis exercisers feel a slight tingling sensation, a sense of itchiness, or a feeling of fatigue (similar to a post-gym workout), whereas others feel nothing. Regardless, your body clues and ruler measurements are much more important than what you feel while stretching. As long as you don't feel any pain, then you are most likely on the right track.

"Can I just stretch straight out?"

You'll want to stretch in every angle possible, not just straight out. Stretching in multiple angles will maximize your growth because stretching in different directions targets different areas. For instance, roughly half of your penis is tucked away inside your body. Many men find that stretching straight down stretches the ligaments, which in turn "releases" some of that tucked away inner penis that's hidden from the outside world.

But you don't want to focus on just stretching down either. By stretching in multiple angles, you're increasing the areas your penis can grow. That's because stretching in other angles also targets different parts of your actual penis. Stretching up actually focuses the stretch on your inner penis; stretching to the right focuses the stretch on the left part of your penis; and stretching left focuses on the right part of your penis. The right and left parts of the penis are known as the corpus chambers and you can learn more about them in Appendix B: The Penis Anatomy.

The only instance that you'll want to stretch in just one direction is if you have a penis curve that you would like to straighten. In this case, focus your stretches in the opposite direction of the curve.

"I can't obtain a good grip when stretching. How do I fix it?"

Use a stretching aide, such as baby powder, rubber gloves, or a fabric of some sort (like a cotton cloth). Baby powder can be placed on your hands and penis; whereas rubber gloves and fabric typically cover your hands. But keep in mind that you shouldn't be pulling too hard. Using too much force too soon can actually impede growth. No matter how hard it is to believe, it is the light and gentle stretches that lead to growth in the beginning.

Basic Stretch Assignment

Do the basic stretch in all directions, twice. This translates into five minutes of basic stretching.

26

The JAI Stretch: Quick & Easy

The basic stretch is just one of fourteen different stretching exercises. Each stretch is similar in form, but unique in the way it places stress on the penis. The JAI stretch is another beginner stretch that you can do whenever you get a few minutes of privacy.

The man who invented this exercise tried every exercise from here to Japan with nothing but failure. He couldn't gain if his sex-life depended on it. But then he applied the concept of active isolated stretching—which involves light, quick stretches—and applied it to penis exercises.[1] The outcome worked so well that he gained within weeks. He's not the only one. Several men report an increase in growth from this exercise.

The best part about JAI stretches is that you don't have to do hundreds for them to work—just do a few here and there. Every time you go to the bathroom, for example. On a thirty second restroom break? Do five to twenty JAI stretches after your done doing your business. You can also use this exercise as a preliminary warm up stretch before you do your other stretches.

The JAI Stretch:

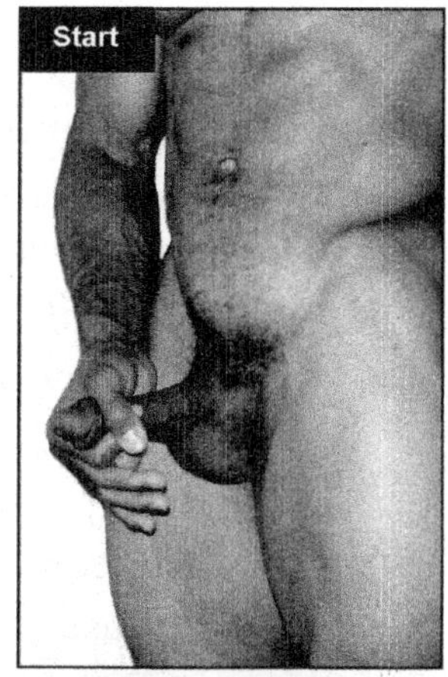

Erection Level: 0 to 40 percent

Recommended Reps for Beginners: 20

The Exercise:

1. Gently stretch your penis and hold for two seconds.
2. Release the stretch for two seconds.
3. Repeat steps one and two until you've completed your desired number of reps.

JAI Stretching Tips!

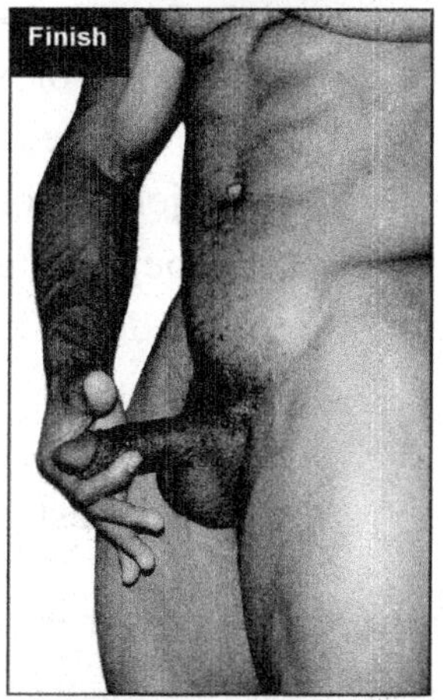

Pattern your breathing:

A great way to get rid of the tedious second counting is to pattern your breathing with your stretch. Do this by exhaling for the two seconds you are pulling out, and inhaling for the two seconds you are resting—or vice versa.

Pull gently:

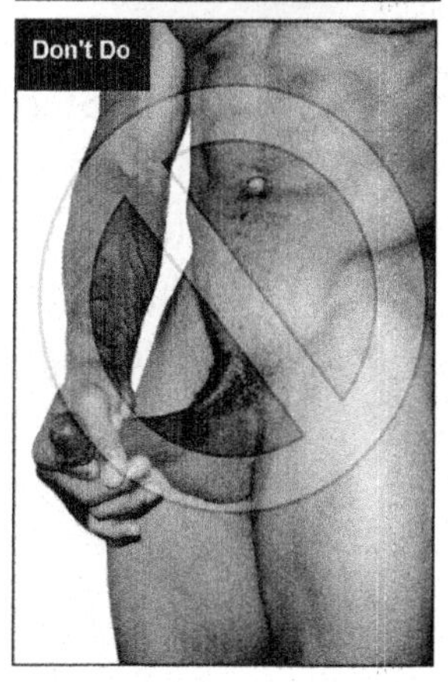

The goal is to perform a light and quick stretch, lasting approximately two seconds. Avoid stretching for more than two seconds. Also, pull slightly lighter than you do with the basic stretch. If you pull too hard, or for too long, the JAI stretches won't be effective. The picture on the right shows the model pulling too hard. Notice how the ligaments at the base of his penis are stretched out and extended much more than in the gentle stretch above (See Appendix B for an illustration of the ligaments).

Part III Review

- ✓ The kegel, unlike other penis exercises, strengthens real skeletal muscles (your pelvic floor muscles).
- ✓ The kegel doesn't require the use of your hands or any other object —only the will of your mind.
- ✓ Kegeling provides an array of benefits for penis enlargement and penis health.
- ✓ Warming up prior to performing penis exercises will enhance gains and reduce injury.
- ✓ Heat increases flexibility and improves blood flow.
- ✓ Exercise immediately after you warm up.
- ✓ Never grip or stroke the head of your penis while performing penis exercises.
- ✓ Avoid jelqing or stretching your penis while it's erect.
- ✓ In the beginning, you'll want to use a lubricant to jelq.
- ✓ Jelqing doesn't require extreme force for it to work; use a light, gentle grip.
- ✓ Ease into stretches and avoid jerking your penis like you're in a tug of war contest.

Important Pages from Part III:

- ➢ Kegel Exercises, page 59
- ➢ Warm Up: Step-by-Step, page 67
- ➢ The Erection Levels, page 78
- ➢ Jelq: Step-by-Step, page 82
- ➢ Basic Stretching: Step-by-Step, page 89
- ➢ JAI Stretching: Step-by-Step, page 92

The First 5 Weeks

Part IV

In this part you will:

- Incorporate the beginner exercises into your first workout routine, which lasts roughly 5 weeks
- Learn how to use the principles from the Circle of Gains in combination with your routine
- Discover more ways to maximize your results
- Learn how to avoid and overcome possible side effects

27

Basic Beginner's Routine

You've learned the basic principles of performing penis exercises. You've learned the beginning exercises. Now it's time to put it together—in the form of a penis exercises routine. In accordance with the basic principles of performing penis exercises, you'll want to start out light and slowly increase the intensity over time. Accordingly, you'll only use the beginning exercises for the first five weeks. Thereafter, you can gradually add more advanced exercises to your workouts.

Similar to gym workout routines, there are countless different penis exercises routines. You can come up with any number of variations by changing the reps you do, the number of days you workout, and the exercises you use. The Basic Beginner's Routine, which incorporates all of the fundamental exercises into a workout, is the most popular beginning routine. This routine is the most effective and is a great starting point for most men. However, if you have fairly weak erections, short-lasting erections, or if you have sex or masturbate less than once a week, then start with one of the alternative routines described in the next chapter, which are less intense.

The Basic Beginner's Routine – 5 Weeks

Three days a week, do the following:

The main workout:

- 10 minute warm up
- 5 minutes of basic stretching
- 10 minutes of jelqing

Anytime throughout the workout day:

- 20 to 60 JAI stretches
- 3 sets of 20 kegels (roughly 1 minute of kegeling)

Everyday:

- Do the kegel start/stop every time you use the restroom

Increase the intensity:

Over five weeks, steadily increase to twenty minutes of jelqing and ten minutes of basic stretching. This is just a suggested guideline, and it's okay if you don't reach this goal. The important thing is that you have healthy body clues and you are gaining.

Add more kegels:

Over five weeks, increase to at least three minutes and no more than five minutes of kegeling per workout. Also, do ten kegel slams once your pelvic floor muscles are strong enough.

When to exercise:

During week 1, take at least two days off between workouts. By week 2, move up to exercising every other day as long as you feel comfortable doing so. By week 3, you can move up to exercising four days a week as long as you have healthy body clues.

Example Calendar for Basic Beginner's Routine

The Basic Beginner's Routine is a guideline. It generally lasts five weeks, but you may need more time. This routine doesn't need to be followed religiously. You are encouraged — and expected — to make it your own. No one knows your penis, your body, and your schedule better than you do. If after five weeks you're ready to increase the intensity even more, proceed to Part V where you can start using advanced exercises.

SUN.	MON.	TUES.	WED.	THURS.	FRI.	SAT.
Workout	Rest Day	Rest Day	**Workout**	Rest Day	Rest Day	**Workout**
Rest Day	**Workout**	Rest Day	**Workout**	Rest Day	**Workout**	Rest Day
Workout	Rest Day	**Workout**	Rest Day	**Workout**	Rest Day	**Workout**
Rest Day	**Workout**	Rest Day	**Workout**	Rest Day	**Workout**	**Workout**
Rest Day	**Workout**	Rest Day	**Workout**	**Workout**	Rest Day	**Workout**

28

Alternative Beginning Routines

Question: "I'm skeptical of exercising my penis, so I'm in no rush. Can I start out with a lighter routine than the Basic Beginner's Routine?"

Yes. There is no set limit on how much—or how little—you exercise. In fact, several men report that they couldn't gain with the basic routine, but when they later switched to a lighter routine they had great results. That's because in the beginning often just a few minutes of performing penis exercises, if done consistently, will encourage growth. Moreover, for some men, the Basic Beginner's Routine is simply too intense.

In this chapter, you will find two other popular beginner routines. Both routines last longer than the traditional five weeks of the Basic Beginner's Routine. Both are also lighter than the Basic Beginner's Routine, so they might be too light for your penis to grow. On the other hand, you may gain even more with one of these routines. It all depends on how "fit" your penis is, your genetics, and other factors.

The Progressive Routine – 8 Weeks

Three days a week, do the following:

The main workout:

- 5 minute warm up
- 2.5 minutes of basic stretching
- 3 minutes of jelqing (75 jelqs)

Continue to do kegels and JAI stretches according to the Basic Beginner's Routine recommendation.

Increase the intensity:

Each week add one minute of jelqing and one minute of stretching.

When to exercise:

During your first week, take at least 2 days off between workouts. By your second week, move up to exercising every other day as long as you feel comfortable doing so. By your third week, you can move up to exercising four days a week as long as you have healthy body clues.

Alternative Routine 1: The Progressive Routine

The Progressive Routine starts light and progressively works its way up. This routine is useful for becoming familiar with performing penis exercises and at the same time making gains with less effort.

Key Points of the Progressive Routine

- Less work than the Basic Beginner's Routine.
- Less chance of over-training or unwanted side effects occurring than with the Basic Beginner's Routine.
- Can be performed quickly in the shower.
- A good starting point for men with weak erections or men who don't use their penis frequently.
- Advance after eight weeks instead of five.
- Growth often doesn't happen as rapidly as the Basic Beginner's Routine.

Example Calendar for Progressive Routine

After eight weeks, move onto Part V and gradually incorporate some advanced exercises into the mix.

SUN.	MON.	TUES.	WED.	THURS.	FRI.	SAT.
Workout	Rest Day	Rest Day	**Workout**	Rest Day	Rest Day	**Workout**
Rest Day	**Workout**	Rest Day	**Workout**	Rest Day	**Workout**	Rest Day
Workout	Rest Day	**Workout**	Rest Day	**Workout**	Rest Day	**Workout**
Rest Day	**Workout**	Rest Day	**Workout**	Rest Day	**Workout**	**Workout**
Rest Day	**Workout**	Rest Day	**Workout**	**Workout**	Rest Day	**Workout**

Alternative Routine 2: The Least Work/Max Gain Routine

The Least Work/Max Gain Routine is best if your time is limited, or if you plan on spending as little time as possible performing penis exercises. The routine was created by a man who uses the online alias Babbis.

In a nutshell, with this routine you perform penis exercises six total days, take a month off, and then repeat. The reason behind the break is simple. Fairly quickly, your penis becomes "conditioned" to the exercises. By taking a break, you're "deconditioning" your penis, and keeping it ready to grow (you'll learn more about conditioning, deconditioning, and breaks in Part V). Numerous penis exercisers report that this light routine makes it easier to stay motivated. Moreover, several beginners find that they gain just as much, in the beginning when using a routine similar to the Least Work/Max Gain Routine.

Key Points of the Least Work/Max Gain Routine

- Maximum amount of growth with least amount of work.
- Less chance of over-training than if were to follow a more intense routine.
- Most men who gain with this routine typically notice results within the first two or three workouts. So if you try this routine, you'll know fairly quickly if it's right for you or not. And if it's not, you can easily switch to the Basic Beginner's Routine.
- Lasts at least eight weeks, and possibly more.
- Isn't as consistent as the Basic Beginner's Routine.
- May not increase hardness as effective as the other routines, largely because of the break. You can counteract this by consistently sticking to a good kegel routine.

The Least Work/Max Gain Routine – 1 to 6 Months

Do the workout, and then rest for 2 days. Do this for a total of 6 workouts (18 total days). Thereafter, do light exercises for 1 week. Then take 1 month off. Continue to do kegels and JAI stretches according to the Basic Beginner's Routine recommendation.

The main workout:

- 10 minute warm up
- 5 minutes of basic stretching
- 7 minutes of jelqing (roughly 150 jelqs)

After the 18 days - Cement, Break, and Repeat:

If you gained using the routine, move onto the 1 week of light exercising and then the break. If you didn't gain, and you don't have unhealthy body clues, proceed to the Basic Beginner's Routine.

1 week of light exercising:

The day after your last main workout, do the following every day for seven days:

- 2.5 minutes of basic stretching (30 second holds in each direction)
- 2 minutes of jelqing (50 jelqs).

1-month break:

During the break, do not do any exercises that actually involve exercising your penis, such as the jelq. Continue to do kegels, and build up their intensity according to the Basic Beginner's Routine.

Repeat:

After the break, repeat the routine as many times as you can gain while doing so. But each time around, add an extra five minutes of jelqing and an extra five minutes of stretching. After three cycles, or when the routine stops providing growth, proceed to Part V and incorporate advanced exercises into the mix.

Example Calendar for Least Work/Max Gain Routine

Measure after every second rest day. If you are still gaining after the sixth workout, continue to exercise every third day until the growth stops. Thereafter, continue to the one week of light exercises. The light exercises serve as a mini-cementing routine to make your gains more likely to be permanent (you'll learn more about cementing and the permanency of gains in Part V).

SUN.	MON.	TUES.	WED.	THURS.	FRI.	SAT.
Workout 1	Rest Day	Rest Day	**Workout 2**	Rest Day	Rest Day	**Workout 3**
Rest Day	Rest Day	**Workout 4**	Rest Day	Rest Day	**Workout 5**	Rest Day
Rest Day	**Workout 6**	**Start of Light Exercise**	*Light Exercise*	*Light Exercise*	*Light Exercise*	*Light Exercise*
Light Exercise	*Light Exercise*	Start Break	**Month-Long Break**			

29

Your Unique Goals

Most penis exercisers share one common goal—the desire for a bigger penis. But their specific goals often differ. Some men want a longer penis as opposed to a thicker one, or vice versa. Some men don't even want a bigger penis; they just want to improve their hardness and their penis health.

Each of these specific goals can be accomplished by following a more specific routine. Follow these guidelines to make your routine more specific.

If You Want Both Length and Girth

Follow the Basic Beginner's Routine or one of the alternative routines from the previous chapter. They have all the key elements of building more girth, more length, and more hardness. Jelqing helps with length, girth, and hardness. Stretching helps with both length and hardness. The kegel is well-known for making the penis harder, but it also makes the penis bigger by increasing penile blood flow.

If You Want Just Length

Focus on both jelqing and stretching. Do your jelqs with a low erection level, around 50 percent. After the first five weeks, add a variety of advanced length exercises and omit the advanced girth exercises. Instead of doing girth exercises, spend the extra time stretching and jelqing.

If You Want Just Girth

For now, focus on jelqing. Do your jelqs with a high erection level, around 75 percent. Also continue to do four or five minutes of stretches before your jelqs, as this keeps the tissues within your penis stretched and ready to expand outward. After the first five weeks, you can start incorporating advanced girth exercises.

If You Want Just Hardness

Follow the Basic Beginner's Routine. Both jelqing and stretching contribute to increased hardness. Also put in an extra effort to do your daily kegels since they are the best exercise for increasing hardness.

If You Want to Straighten a Curve

Penis exercising has helped several men straighten a curve in their penis, mainly with exercises that are focused on going "against the curve." You can learn how to incorporate curve-fixing exercises into your routine in Appendix A, under the section "Fixing a Penis Curve."

30

Your Unique Penis

The Basic Beginner's Routine has all the crucial elements of a successful workout plan. Still, this routine may not fit everyone's individual needs for growth. That's because there isn't such a thing as a magic, one-size-fits-all routine. And for this reason, the Basic's Beginner's Routine is just a general guideline. Routines similar to it have worked for thousands of men, but it still may be too intense—or maybe even too light—for you. Every man's penis is different. Not all penises are as *physically* fit as one another, nor are they the same *anatomically.*

From the anatomy standpoint, an example of how each man's penis is different involves the tunica—a tissue that surrounds the penis just beneath the skin. The tunica is a multi-layered, tendon-like tissue that governs the size of the penis. It is extremely strong. Most penises have two layers of tunica. Some penises, however, have only one layer of tunica; others have three.[1] It has been suggested that perhaps men gain quicker (or slower) depending on how many layers of tunica they have. Regardless, the unique anatomy of your penis and your genetics will presumably play a crucial part in how your penis reacts to certain exercises and routines, and ultimately how much your penis grows.

Just as important as the anatomy of your penis—and possibly even more important—is the fitness level of your penis. That is, *how physically fit is your penis*? How often is your penis put to work? How often do you get an erection, masturbate, or have sex?

A man who masturbates or has sex only once or twice a week has a less physically fit penis than a man who has sex daily. Similarly, a man whose average sex session is no more than ten minutes has a weaker penis than a man who typically has sex for an hour or more. Simply put, a man who uses his penis more has a more physically fit penis.

These two differences—anatomy and fitness—can cause problems with a set routine. For instance, a man with a weak penis may find that Basic's Beginner's Routine is too intense for him. Or a man with a strong, fit penis may find that the Basic Beginner's Routine is not intense enough.

For comparison, it's easy to find out what works for you while exercising at the gym. You lift the highest amount of weight possible, or "max out," and then base your workouts off that weight. Because there is no way to find your max when performing penis exercises, you may be going way beyond your max and over-training, or way below it and under-training—and therefore stopping yourself from gaining without even knowing it.

Let's say, for example, that you're bench pressing and your max is 200 pounds. But let's pretend you don't know your max. You're exercising in the dark. You start out lifting only fifty pounds for a few weeks, but this isn't enough weight to cause any growth (you're under-training). So you decide to bump it up a notch and lift 300 pounds (which is way past over-training). Not only do you not grow, but you also have a broken rib cage from dropping the weight on your chest.

This is exactly what is going on when you perform penis exercises—you're exercising "in the dark." Fortunately, there is one way to combat this in the dark exercising, and it involves that all-important principle of performing penis exercises.

The most important thing you can do is pay attention to your body clues—they are more important than any set number of reps, time, or routine. As you know, your body clues let you know when to increase the intensity and when to step back.

As you advance, use the body clue cheat sheet, in Chapter 11, along with the general guideline below to help direct you:

- * If you have **healthy** body clues and you are **gaining**, then you are on the right track.
- If you have **healthy** body clues—or no clear indication of unhealthy body clues—**and you are not gaining**, then you are most likely not using enough intensity. Gradually bump it up until you start gaining.
- If you have **unhealthy** body clues and you are **not gaining**, then you need more rest and less intensity.

31

Putting the Circle of Gains into Practice

Now that you are exercising your penis, let's dig up those all-important principles form the Circle of Gains—*obtain adequate rest*, *increase the intensity*, and *pay attention to your body clues*—and demonstrate how easily they fit into your routine. To do this, here's a profile of a typical penis exerciser. Let's call him Billy.

Scenario 1

Billy starts off using the Basic Beginner's Routine. He makes sure to get at least two days of rest between workouts. After one week, Billy notices stronger erections and more erections throughout the night—two healthy body clues. Billy continues with the routine. After two more days, Billy's erections are still harder and more frequent. On top of that, he measures a gain of .125 inches in both length and girth.

Billy knows he is on the right track because he is experiencing all healthy body clues along with the best clue of them all—growth. At this point, Billy can go in two directions. He can either continue with his current routine until the growth stops, or he can gradually increase the intensity in an effort to keep growth coming in steady.

Billy decides to gradually add more time to his workout. Over the next two weeks he adds an additional minute of jelqing to each workout day. By the end of the second week, he is jelqing for an extra six minutes. He is also exercising every other day. Billy's routine looks like this:

The End of Week 3:

- 10 minute warm up
- 5 minutes of basic stretching
- 16 minutes of jelqing

This goes well for Billy, as he gains another .125" length. Keep in mind that Billy didn't just add six minutes to his jelqing routine. He added one minute of jelqing to every workout day. This gradual build up—opposed to a giant leap—is what separates growth from over-training

Scenario 2

After four weeks, Billy is performing penis exercises four days a week. He still makes an effort to get at least one day of rest between most of his workouts. His kegels are also up to three minutes each workout day. To make things easy, he breaks the kegeling sessions into three, one minute sessions. He does one minute in the morning, one in the afternoon, and one in the evening.

Everything is going well for Billy. He has made continual gains and has yet to experience an unhealthy body clue. In light of his success, Billy believes his penis can handle much more than he is giving it. So, in an effort to speed up the growth, Billy decides to add ten extra minutes of jelqing and ten extra minutes of stretching. His routine now looks like this:

The Beginning of Week 5:

- 10 minute warm up
- 15 minutes of basic stretching
- 26 minutes of jelqing

After a week, Billy starts noticing negative changes. Billy experiences numbness after his workouts, weaker erections, and a smaller flaccid penis—three unhealthy body clues. And he hasn't gained.

The unhealthy body clues indicate that Billy is most likely over-training By rapidly upping his workout, Billy went well over his "max." Although performing penis exercises forty minutes per workout after four weeks is okay for a few men, it's clearly too much for Billy.

Everybody is different, and this is why the body clues are the most important aspect of performing penis exercises—they guide your routine. In this case, Billy's body clues are telling him to hit the brakes, slow down, and take a step back.

Scenario 3

To recuperate from his over-training, Billy makes it an effort to give his penis rest. He wisely waits for his erections to return to normal before jumping back into the swing of things. When Billy returns, he goes back to the last routine in which he was experiencing healthy body clues. Going back to the last routine where things were good and healthy is often the best place to restart when things go bad. Billy is back to using this routine:

Week 6:

- 10 minute warm up
- 5 minutes of basic stretching
- 16 minutes of jelqing

Billy's initial five weeks are complete, so he can technically (but definitely shouldn't) advance past the beginner routine and use some advance exercises. But Billy knows that he's not ready just yet. He just got over a big set-back. For this reason, Billy continues to use the same routine for the next few workouts.

Fairly quickly, Billy starts to experience healthy body clues again. He isn't gaining though, so he decides to increase the intensity. Over the next two weeks, he finishes the Basic Beginner's Routine recommendations, and his routine now looks like this:

Week 8:

- 10 minute warm up
- 10 minutes of basic stretching
- 20 minutes of jelqing

This works well for Billy, as he gains .25" in length and .125" in girth. Now that Billy is ready to move up—which is evident by his healthy body clues—he proceeds to the Basic Advancing Routine (outlined in Part V).

Adding it Up

On the surface, it might seem as if Billy wasn't gaining much—just a little bit here and there. But these small gains add up. Over the long haul, Billy gained half an inch in length and a quarter an inch in girth. For an average-sized penis, this is roughly a 15 percent increase in volume. In practice, this is how performing penis exercises works. You gain in small increments, and overtime those increments convert to extra inches on the ruler.

32

Maximizing Gains

Along with sticking to the basic principles like a magnet to a refrigerator, there are several other ways you can maximize your growth. Follow the thirteen tips below to get the best out of your workouts.

1 – Finish Each Workout With a Healthy Erection

If you can't get an erection at the end of your workout—and you typically have healthy erections—then you over-trained during that particular workout. Next time use more rest and less intensity. A penile workout should leave your penis rejuvenated, not exhausted.

2 – Add Masturbation

Many men find that adding masturbation to the mix not only helps boost their gains but also helps build stamina in the bedroom. So, if you have the time, masturbate for a few minutes before or after your routine. Especially focus on staying close to the edge of ejaculation, as your penis is biggest right before you ejaculate. "I always edge after I exercise my penis," says one man who added nearly four inches to his penis. "I started out only being able to do it for 10 to 15 minutes, but I got better. Now I edge for 60 minutes and release my load every third workout. I do that because I feel like your penis exercising session is that much better if you don't climax your edge."

You also don't want to masturbate too much. Masturbating can have a negative effect on your gains, depending on how long you do it, the amount of intensity you use, and the ability of your penis to recover. For example, if a man masturbates for several hours (this happens), it can be as much or more stress to his penis as an actual penis exercises workout. The only way you can tell if masturbating is beneficial or harmful to your gains is to pay close attention to your body clues afterward.

Also, whether you ejaculate or not is up to you. A lot of penis exercisers believe that not ejaculating two hours before or after a workout maximizes gains. The argument for this belief is that you want your penis to be relaxed, full of blood, and larger than normal after a penis exercises workout. And you've probably noticed that the penis often contracts, shrinks, and reduces in blood flow after ejaculation. Nevertheless, several men have gained inches regardless of when they ejaculated. In the end, if you want to ejaculate, go for it. If after a while you feel that ejaculating is hurting your gains, try holding off ejaculating for two hours before and after your routine to see if it helps.

3 – Practice Proper Technique

The chief reason some men can't gain is improper technique. Bad technique includes jerking stretches and using an improper grip while jelqing. Penis exercises are easy to do, yet they may take a few attempts to master. To make sure you have the technique down, use the pictures and descriptions of the exercises the first few times you do them. Also, for a better understanding, watch the "how-to" videos of the exercises at http://www.PEGym.com.

4 – Pain = No Gain

One major difference between exercising the muscles and exercising the penis is the popular gym motto: No Pain = No Gain. Several people feel that if you don't feel pain while working out, you're not going to gain. This is often untrue, and it's even more untrue when performing penis exercises.

Penis exercising with the pain-is-good mentality will cause nothing but harm. In fact, if you ever think you're going at it too intensely, then you probably are. Listen to your body, it rarely steers you wrong. When exercising the penis I want you to adapt a new motto: Pain = No Gain! If you feel pain or a lack of sensation, stop immediately.

5 – Remember Your Kegels

A big pitfall for beginners is forgetting—or purposely avoiding—the kegel. Men are especially prone to skipping the kegel during the first few weeks, when it's easy to get wrapped up in the other fundamental exercises.

Kegels are an important part of any penis exercises routine. They are indispensable for hardness and your overall penis health, and they can also help with penis enlargement growth by increasing blood flow. Moreover, kegels are an easy and mindless task, so why skip them. Always do the kegel start/stop. It's a simple exercise that requires a few extra seconds of doing something you will already be doing—urinating.

6 – Always Warm up

A warm up is essential to healthy penis exercises. I've found that many times when a man isn't gaining, he is either warming up improperly or not warming up at all. Take the case of a penis exerciser who uses the online alias Shiver. Like many other penis exercisers, he never did a warm up because "it didn't seem to be the 'meat' of the program." Shiver had been performing penis exercises for several years (on and off) with only a small gain to show for it, so he decided to investigate what was going wrong. After some research, he learned the importance of heat when stretching tissue. Within two weeks of applying a warm up, Shiver gained nearly a half an inch in length, which is more than he had gained in all his previous years of performing penis exercises.

A warm up should make your penis more elastic than normal. If this isn't happening, you aren't acquiring sufficient heat. In which case, try switching your warm up method, or warm up for longer periods of time.

7 – Cool Down After Each Workout

For one reason or another, some men "warm up" after a workout in hopes they'll increase the benefits that heat provides. This isn't recommended. A chief reason the warm up is so important is that it increases the elasticity of your penis. Increased elasticity, however, is not what you want at the end of your workout. Post workout, the goal is to keep your penis in an enlarged and stretched state. Applying heat to your penis counteracts this goal.

Instead of applying heat to your penis after a workout, try applying cold. Many men find that it helps boost gains and keep the penis in a stretched state. For a cool down, apply cold to your penis using a cold wash cloth, a cold pack that has been sitting in the fridge (not the freezer), or some cold water. Keep the cool down applied for one to two minutes. Just make sure it's not too cold, or your penis is liable to contract and shrink up.

8 – Do JAI Stretches

The JAI stretch may look minor and ineffective, but it's far from it. Time after time, men have told me that they didn't start gaining until they added JAI stretches into the mix. Many men find that doing twenty or more JAI stretches before and after their routine helps, along with doing ten or so every time they use the restroom.

9 – Learn From Your Mistakes

If you know that a certain exercise or routine isn't working, then try something different. At first, knowing what works and what doesn't will seem like guesswork. But as time goes on, you will become completely in sync with your penis. As one penis exerciser who uses the online alias Peter Dick says, "It's possible for almost anyone to gain . . . providing they perform penis exercises the right way." Peter Dick never hit a plateau—in which growth comes to a halt—and gained nearly two and half inches. How did he do it? He says, "I'm very in tune with my dick, and I know what works for me."

10 – Don't Beat Yourself Up If You Don't Gain Right Away

Getting into the groove takes time, and impatience is the downfall for many men. Some men go several months—and sometimes much longer—without gaining. And then, through trial and error, they suddenly start gaining.

Enlarging your penis isn't an instantaneous process. As Tom Hubbard, a man who helped lay the foundation of the modern penis exercises community, says, "Rome wasn't built in a day. Neither is a new penis." Change for the better takes time. Be consistent, keep at it, and the gains will come.

11 – Don't Move Up Too Fast

I know, I know, you get it—but this point cannot be stressed enough. It's ironic: there's a fine line between over-training (using too much intensity) and under-training (not using enough intensity). Between that line is where you want to be: gaining. Although both under-training and over-training can stop you from gaining, it's much better to be under-training

The worst thing you can do is start out using too much intensity, as over-training can be discouraging. The main indication of over-training is weaker erections. And if your penis has a weak erection at the wrong time —say when your partner is ready to put in the Marvin Gaye CD and "get it on"—then you're liable to swear off penis exercises for good.

Even worse, several men notice that when they continually over-train by moving up too fast, it makes it even harder for them to gain in the future. That's because the penis adapts and gets tougher each time you over-train So moving up too fast is a double-edge sword: Not only does it stop you from gaining now, but also in the future. The best way to avoid this problem is to start out light—perhaps even under-train at first—and increase the intensity as necessary.

If you're ever in doubt about when to up the intensity, then don't do it. After the doubt subsides, move forward with caution. Don't let your wants replace your needs. Your penis needs adequate rest and proper conditioning.

The Other Side of the Story: Not Increasing the Intensity

Although I recommend in this book that you should continue to gradually increase the intensity overtime (as long as you have healthy body clues!), some men find that it's safer to not increase the intensity until gains have come to a complete halt. Following this method, you would stick with a fairly similar routine until you have gained all you can using that routine, and then increase the intensity until you start gaining again. The best part about this method is that it's a lot easier to avoid going overboard this way.

12 – Track Your Progress in a Journal

Along with providing continual motivation, a progress journal will allow you to record your workouts and your gains. By tracking your results and what you did to obtain those results, you will know exactly how your penis responds to certain exercises and routines.

Every now and then, you can review your progress journal and see if you can find a pattern. For example, you might notice that you experience your best gains when you give your penis two days of rest between workouts. You don't have to track your progress each workout, but I suggest that you do it roughly every week or so. The more often you track your results, the more accurate your progress journal will be.

In Appendix D, I have provided a progress journal sheet for you. You can either make photocopies of the page, or you can find the same page on the companion website to this book, http://www.PEGym.com/progress and print it from there. Make several copies and put them into a penis exercises binder.

If you don't want to keep a progress journal on paper, you can take the next step and track your results online. In fact, if you're able, I recommend that you track your progress on Internet support forums, as others can critique your routines, methods, and other variables that you haven't considered. You can start a progress journal in the community forums at one of the recommended websites in Appendix D.

At http://www.PEGym.com, you can also find several tools that make it easy to record your progress online and get feedback in the progress blogs section.

In your progress journal, list the exercises used, the degree of intensity applied, and the amount of time spent performing penis exercises on each exercise. For even better accuracy, also list your warm-up method, the amount of time you spent warming up, and any additional notes that you find beneficial. Some men, for example, also list the supplements, vitamins, and medications they took that week to help determine everything that might affect growth. The more information you provide, the greater chance you 'll repeat good results.

13 – Try Different Variations

Different alterations of exercises and routines work for different men. For example, as a general rule, jelqing with a lower erection level builds length and a higher erection level builds girth. But a few men have reported that jelqing with a higher erection level helped them build length, and others reported that jelqing with a lower erection level helped them build girth. So, although I can lay the groundwork for you by giving you the general rules, only you will be able to find out what works best for you. You can do this by keeping it varied, trying new things, and tracking your results as you progress.

33

Overcoming Possible Side Effects & Minor Setbacks

"The penis is mightier than the sword."

-Mark Twain

With the right training, penis exercises are as healthy for your penis as running is for your heart. Thousands of men have already made their penises bigger, harder, and healthier with the methods described in this book. So can you.

You, as many men before you, can reap the rewards of penis exercises. But just as running might cause leg cramps and sore joints, penis exercises might also bring about unwanted bumps in the road. These minor setbacks, which are often just negative side effects, could set you back anywhere from a day to a week or more. Most side effects are small and clear up in just a few days—for instance, little red bumps caused by overexertion, or dry skin as a result of a bad reaction to a lubricant.

Sometimes side effects aren't even side effects. The "problem" may have been there all along. One man, for example, was frightened because he found a small bump on the underside of his penis. He was sure jelqing caused it. Then when he showed the bump to his wife, she exclaimed, "That little bump? You've had that for over ten years!" This chapter isn't meant to scare you. It's meant to prepare you. In fact, it's possible that you won't encounter one side effect. If you do, odds are that it will either be slight darkening or little red spots. Nevertheless, you should be aware of the side effects that are possible. This chapter will go over both the common and the rare side effects that other penis exercisers have endured, and what to do if they occur, including:

- Pain
- A darker penis
- Bruises
- Spotting along the penis
- The doughnut effect
- Dry skin
- Blisters
- Blood
- Thrombosed vein (or penile Mondor's disease)
- Temporary erectile dysfunction

Pain is Bad

Remember that pain is the ultimate unhealthy body clue. Pain, by nature, is never good. So if in any instance you experience pain, stop what you are doing—it will almost always go away without further ado. If the pain persists, try using warm wraps, cold wraps, and gentle massages.

Warm Wraps

Heat generally provides pain relief. Warm wraps include your typical warm up methods: a moist heating pad, a heated gel pack, a hot wash cloth, a rice sock, or anything else that applies heat to your penis.

Cold Wraps

Cold, for many, relieves pain better than heat does. When pain occurs, many men find that cold wraps are good for the initial treatment, and a combination of hot and cold is best for further treatment. Regardless, neither heat nor cold should be constantly applied to the penis. Instead, as many medical professionals recommend, rotate between cold for twenty minutes, heat for twenty minutes, and gentle massages for ten or so minutes. In any regard, it's unlikely the pain will last for more than a few seconds, let alone an hour. If it does last anywhere near that long—and it's not just minor soreness—then see a doctor immediately.

Gentle Massages

It's hard to believe that a little tender, love, and care has such a profound effect on your penis. But this antidote plays a significant role in decreasing the extent of several side effects, including pain itself. It comes as no surprise that the penis—an organ that reacts positively to touch—benefits from gentle massages.

The Side Effects

Side effects can be positive or negative. An obvious positive effect is an increase in size. Negative side effects can range from darkening to dry skin. In this chapter, I'm only going to focus on the negative side effects, and what other penis exercisers have done to conquer them (I'll let you decide how to use your positive side effects).

Side Effect: A Darker Penis

A common, yet often preventable, side effect is darkening of the penis. Commonly known as "discoloration" in the penis exercises community, this side effect has had mixed reviews. Some men love the look. As one penis exerciser reflected, "It makes my penis look manlier and less child-like." Other men detest the darker look, especially if they're one of the few men who experienced a more extreme and unusual darkening effect, which is often described as a "long-lasting skin staining."

The Cause

A darker penis is generally caused by intensely performing penis exercises, over-training, or not obtaining an adequate warm up. It is clearly associated with intense exercises—often advanced girth exercises and penis enlargement devices. The extreme and rare "skin-staining" type of darkening that a few men experience is almost always caused by using too much intensity with a device, generally a clamping device. Either way, it's clear that some men are more prone to discoloration than others. Just as some men bruise easily, some men darken easily too. A few unfortunate men experience the darkening effect after doing any penis exercise, no matter how light it is. On the other hand, several men never warm up, use exceedingly intense exercises, and notoriously over-train, yet still experience no darkening whatsoever.

What to Do

Post-workout redness, red spots, and skin flush are normal and shouldn't cause too much alarm. If, however, skin flush and red spots almost always occur, then it could possibly turn into the longer-lasting darkening that most men don't like. Luckily, several penis exercisers have found ways around the darkening effect. If you want to avoid darkening and it starts to become a problem for you, try the following:

Use more heat:

A thorough warm up is crucial, and makes all the difference. A warm wash cloth isn't as effective as a warm up that continually applies the same amount of heat, such as a moist heating pad. Also, try warming up longer and using more heat throughout your workout. Every ten minutes, for example, reapply a warm up for a minute or two. Adding more heat to your workouts is often all it takes to dissipate the darkening effect. As one penis exerciser put it, "I use to have a real bad problem with discoloration, and then I dedicated more time to warming up and haven't had any problems since."

Use gentle massages:

Many men find that gentle massages—especially when combined with heat—reduces the darkening effect.

Use less force:

The darkening effect is most likely caused by trauma to the skin, often by using too much force. So try a more subtle, gentle approach when performing penis exercises. Use less force when stretching and jelqing, and avoid the intense exercises that cause the most darkening for you. For many men, this means avoiding the dry jelq.

Also avoid intense pressure build up with jelqs and girth exercises. A man who uses the online alias Hobby, and who has had his fair share of darkening, suggests, "I think a key way to avoid discoloration, or at least not to intensify it, is to avoid building pressure under tightly stretched skin."

Change your lubricant:

If you don't already, try using a more skin-friendly lubricant, such as baby oil with aloe and vitamin E. Olive oil and canola oil have proven to be easy on the skin too.

Exercise your entire penis:

One major complaint about darkening is that for some men the penis only darkens in certain areas. If this is a problem for you, make sure you are exercising your entire penis. For example, be sure to do full jelqs: start from the very base of your penis and stop right before the head. Also avoid continually gripping the same exact place when stretching. One penis exerciser found that he only experienced discoloration in the area where he gripped. He eventually overcame this by constantly gripping in different points along the shaft—the base, mid-shaft, and right below the head.

Apply cream:

Some penis exercisers have had success with applying Arnica cream, Vitamin K cream, or skin lightening cream to the darkened areas.

One of these creams—if not all—should be available at your local pharmacy, health food store, or department store. They are often found in the cosmetics department. Your best bet is most likely a Vitamin K and Arnica combined cream, such as the one made by Vita-K Solution.

If all else fails, take a break:

The darkening effect often fades with time. Many times it will go away as quickly as weeks. Yet, in severe cases, it takes months, and even years, for the penis to return to its normal color. If the darkening effect becomes a problem, take a few weeks off and see if the problem fades. Either way, the darkening effect rarely happens overnight. It's generally a slow process. So if you notice it taking place and you don't like it, immediately conquer it. Avoid waiting until it's already happened and you should be able to overcome this side effect.

Side Effect: Bruises

Sometimes the penis becomes darker in certain spots, which could be a secluded kind of darkening. On the other hand, it could be a bruise.

The Cause

"Bruises may look nasty and hurt like crazy, but they're really no big deal, says Bill Gottlied in New Choices in Natural Healing. "Any time you bump into something sharp or take a fall, you're likely to develop one. They get their telltale color from blood that pools under the skin after you break a blood vessel." If a bruise does occur in association with performing penis exercises, it's a major clue that you're going overboard with the intensity.

What to Do

Recall that bruising is an unhealthy body clue. So, first and foremost, take a break from performing penis exercises. Let your penis return to normal before you start performing penis exercises again. From there, either leave it alone completely, or find other remedies to help move things along. For example, Richard Gerson, Ph.D., author of The Right Vitamins, says, "To speed up the healing process, I recommend taking 5,000 milligrams of vitamin C at the earliest sign of a bruise." To also help with a speedy recovery, other nutritionists suggest taking daily supplements of vitamin A and E. An additional common therapy involves applying arnica cream, which is a common herbal medicine used for the relief of bruises, stiffness, and muscle soreness. "Arnica erases bruises by helping the body reabsorb the blood that has seeped into tissues. A cream or ointment containing 5% to 25% arnica extract, applied several times daily, reduces pain and swelling—along with that ugly eggplant color," says The Editors of Reader's Digest in their book 1,801 Home Remedies.

After the bruise disappears, start back up with a more gentle approach. Use less force. Depending on where the bruise formed, you might have used too much force on a particular part of the shaft. For example, if the bruise formed on the underside of your penis or on the head of the penis, then you jelqed or griped the underside of your penis with too much pressure. In this case, use a pincher grip in the future when stretching and jelqing. A pincher grip puts less pressure on the underside of your penis, and more pressure on the sides of your penis.

Side Effect: Spotting Along the Penis

When you first start performing penis exercises, spots—medically known as petechiae—might form on the penis. They often form on the head of the penis. Spots are fairly common in the beginning. They generally range anywhere from one to a dozen, and shouldn't cause any worry. They usually clear up in a day or two. The spots are normally red in color, but occasionally come in darker colors (purple and black). Generally, the darker the spots, the more time your penis will need to heal.

The Cause

Spots typically form as a reaction to the new stress of performing penis exercises, most often jelqing. Prior to performing penis exercises, the penis is typically not submitted to a great deal of pressure. Once you start performing penis exercises, the stress of the jelq and other exercises often cause the untouched capillaries underneath the skin to bruise. If you're susceptible to spots, they will most likely occur less and less as time goes on. In the future, the spots might show up after using high intensity exercises, or when returning to a high intensity routine after some time off. The spots do not usually affect growth or hardness. Nevertheless, if they constantly form as a result of excessive intensity, then ease up. You don't want to cause a more serious problem in the future. Persistently spotting can also increase the darkening effect.

Neutral Body Clues

Question: "My penis spots after a workout. Is this an unhealthy body clue?"

For some men, spots form on the penis after an effective, healthy workout. For other men, it's a clear sign of over-training For this reason, spotting isn't an unhealthy body clue, nor is it a healthy body clue. It's more like a neutral body clue. Meaning, you have to interpret it in relation to your gains and the other body clues you are experiencing. For example, if your penis grows with the spots, it's probably a healthy body clue for you. On the other hand, if your penis doesn't grow, it's probably an unhealthy body clue. Other common "neutral" body clues include redness, darkening, and turtling—in which your penis contracts like a turtle's head into its shell right after a workout (not to be confused with decreased flaccid size throughout the entire day—an unhealthy body clue).

What to Do

If you experience unhealthy body clues, or no clear indication of healthy body clues, then avoid performing penis exercises until the spots go away. If you experience healthy body clues along with the spots, then you can continue with your workouts.

Either way, the spots should disappear after a couple of days. To speed up the process, try applying warm wraps, cold wraps, and gentle massages throughout the day. If the spots continue to get worse, leave your penis alone (no penis exercises, masturbation, or sex) until they dissipate. If the spots continually form on the head of your penis because of jelqing, switch to the pincher grip.

Side Effect: The Doughnut Effect

A penis exerciser who uses the alias BoardLurker on the online penis exercises community Thunder's Place describes the doughnut effect best: "There you are jelqing, and all of a sudden your penis looks like the stay-puff marshmallow man! What happened? Odds are, it's the doughnut effect and you have just pushed too much fluid into your penis. This usually looks as it's described; like you have a doughnut on the end of your penis."

The Cause

The doughnut effect is normally associated with jelqing, but it also might occur after long sessions of masturbation or sex. It typically occurs when you force an excessive amount of fluid and blood towards the head of your penis.

What to Do

The doughnut effect generally doesn't last long. Most men only endure it for a few minutes. For some men, however, the doughnut effect can last for a few hours or more. Regardless, it will almost always go away if you leave it alone. To speed up the process, gently massage the doughnut until it dissipates.

Side Effect: Dry Skin

Every once in a while, a man reports that the skin on his penis turns dry and in some instances starts to shed. "Skin shedding" is fairly rare — but if the skin on the penis becomes extremely dry, like any other body part, it might shed.

The Cause

If dry skin is a result of performing penis exercises, it most likely has to do with your lubrication, generally through an allergic reaction to an ingredient in the lubricant. Also, for one reason or another, many men have had bad experiences with lotion or soap as a lubricant. Dry skin can also be caused by lack of lubrication. Dry jelqing, for instance, can produce abrasion along the skin, which occasionally causes the skin to go dry and shed.

What to Do

If you believe your lubricant is causing the problem, change it. Baby oil or Vaseline rarely causes any trouble. If you've been dry jelqing or using little lubrication, then use more in the future.

Side Effect: Blisters

Blisters in relation to performing penis exercises are rare.

The Cause

Blisters are more often associated with a Sexually Transmitted Disease (STD), particularly genital herpes, than with penis exercises. Yet, every now and then, penis exercises might bring about a blister—for example, if you accidentally pinch your penis with your hands or a device.

What to Do

If it is a single blister, which you believe to be caused by something minor—such as a skin pinch—then avoid penis exercises until the blister heals. If the blisters persist, go to the doctor. Get tested for an STD. In a study conducted at Emory University, the authors report, "Each year in the United States, roughly 4 million new sexually transmitted disease infections are diagnosed."[1] That's not including the sexual diseases that aren't diagnosed. In short, it's better to know now than to be sorry about it later. When it comes to sexually transmitted diseases, the quicker you initiate treatment, the better your chance of keeping the damage to a minimum.

Side Effect: Blood

Blood in association with penis exercises is also rare. When blood does occur, it is usually just a couple of drops near the head of the penis. The blood is typically near (or comes out of) the urethra—the canal from which urine and semen are discharged. Sometimes blood is also forced out of the thin skin covering the head of the penis.

The Cause

If blood is coming out of your urethra, the distress could be completely unrelated to penis exercises. It could also be much more serious, especially if you notice blood in your urine, which could be a variety of problems.

Harris H. McIlwain, M.D., who has been twice named one of the Best Doctors in America by Town and Country, says, "Causes of blood in the urine include kidney stones, kidney diseases, bladder diseases (such as cancer), prostate diseases, urinary tract infections, and other medical problems. In all cases, whether the blood is present in large or small amounts, a thorough evaluation is needed."

If a doctor visit indicates nothing serious is wrong, then it may just be a case of too much pressure building up inside the penis. The intense pressure could be caused by using too intense of a grip when jelqing, or too much intensity in general. It could also be caused by vigorous sex or masturbation.

What to Do

First, seek medical attention. As the renowned Dr. Drew of Loveline suggests, "You should always get checked out by a doctor if you experience blood coming out of the penis."

If it is a severe problem, it needs to be addressed right away. If the doctor indicates nothing serious is wrong, give your penis rest. Take a week off from performing penis exercises to allow the problem to heal. Don't jump back into exercising your penis, or you're likely to add fuel to the fire. In the meantime, try rotating between warm wraps, cold wraps, and gentle massages. Once you return to performing penis exercises, use less intensity.

Side Effect: Thrombosed Vein

Bigger, healthier veins are a fairly common side effect of performing penis exercises. Occasionally, however, a penis exerciser reports that he has a thrombosed penile vein. Meaning, the vein is clotted and inflamed, which is medically known as penile Mondor's disease and generally lasts four to six weeks.[2] The disease is rare. "Mondor's disease of the penis is an uncommon condition," says Dr. Mauro Dicuio and colleagues in a study published in the Archive of Italian Urology and Andrology. Penile Mondor's was discovered in 1958, and since then "around fifty cases have been reported."

The chief symptom of penile Mondor's disease is described as a persistent "cord or string-like" firmness along a vein. Other common symptoms include the vein being red, swollen, hot, and hard. Sometimes mild pain is a symptom too. If you experience most of these symptoms—especially a vein that is hardened, red-colored, and exerted—you should be alarmed, but not worried. It's most likely just bigger, more prominent penile veins—not penile Mondor's.

But if you do have penile Mondor's disease, which is unlikely but possible, the good news is that it usually lasts no more than two to eight weeks. Moreover, as Dr. Mauro Dicuio and colleagues note, penile Mondor's is "benign"—meaning it isn't harmful to your body, nor is it harmful to the long-term use of your penis. As another study declared, "there is no report of erectile dysfunction after treatment." Even so, immediately stop doing whatever caused the clotted vein so it doesn't turn into anything more serious.

The Cause

Penile Mondor's disease is often associated with vigorous or excessive sexual activity. So it makes sense that vigorous penis exercises might also bring about the disease. In fact, the majority of penis exercisers who have shown similar symptoms of penile Mondor's disease were using excessive amounts of intensity, often with a penis enlargement device. This is another reason why you'll want to start light and work your way up.

But vigorous penis exercises and sex may not be the predominating cause. After all, millions of men partake in sex that is vigorous and haven't had the slightest problem. So is there another cause for the disease? Some doctors think so.

In a study published in *The Journal of the American Osteopathic Association*, Dr. David Griger and colleagues point out, "Many predisposing factors can lead to the development of penile Mondor's disease… which all relate back to vessel wall damage, stasis, and a state in which clots easily form." If you combine vigorous penis exercises or vigorous sex with these factors, you might just have a recipe for penile Mondor's disease.

Either way, in the future you should avoid whatever initially clotted the vein. As Dr. Griger and colleagues indicate, "evidence suggests that men who acquire penile Mondor's disease once are predisposed to having recurrent episodes."

His Story

A Happy Ending

A penis exerciser who uses the online name ManChuck would occasionally have an enlarged vein that was red, hot, hard, and painful, and in all likelihood a form of penile Mondor's disease. He reported that for the past five years—long before he started performing penis exercises—the enlarged, painful vein would last anywhere from a week to three months. In the past year he finally found his remedy: take baby aspirin every day.

What to Do

First and foremost, those who experience Mondor's disease should abstain from penis exercises, sex, and masturbation until the problem subsides. The best thing any man can do in the instance of penile Mondor's disease is leave his penis alone. The longer the problem is ignored, the more recovery time will be needed.

It's also recommended that you go see a doctor if you believe you have penile Mondor's disease. An experienced physician will be able to do a Doppler scan and other tests to see if the condition is in fact a thrombosed vein.

Several urologists suggest taking 400 milligrams of Ibuprofen, three times daily for the first week of penile Mondor's disease, as it often speeds up the healing process. Some men have also found that Essential Vein Oil (EVO) and other lubricants created specifically for penis exercises work well in quickly relieving penile Mondor's disease. The creator of EVO, a penis exerciser who uses the online alias Eroset, suggests massaging the affected vein with EVO for five to ten minutes, two to three times a day. Eroset also suggests leaving the EVO on your penis (unless you experience skin irritation), because "your penis will continue to absorb the oils after your massage if you leave it on." For instructions on how to make EVO, see Appendix D: Penis Exercising Resources. To find other pre-made lubricants with vasodilators, go to http://www.PEGym.com/penis-lubricants.

Some men also advocate rotating warm wraps, cold wraps, and gentle slow massages to influence (not force) the vein to unclot. Any of these methods might help you speed up the process and alleviate the pain, in the instance that penile Mondor's disease occurs. Again, penile Mondor's disease is rare; and most of the time when a man thinks he has thrombosed a vein in his penis, he usually just has bigger, more visible penile veins.

Side Effect: Temporary Erectile Dysfunction

Erectile dysfunction — the inability to maintain an erection—is a clear sign that you're over-training This is based on the assumption that you had healthy erections prior to performing penis exercises.

The Cause

Temporary erectile dysfunction is usually a sign of an exhausted penis. Think of your penis as any other muscle; it can only take so much stress before it becomes flimsy and nearly unusable. That's why you might notice a weaker erection right after a marathon sex session—your penis is exhausted (although it's common to notice stronger erections after the healing process kicks in).

What to Do

Anything related to poor erection quality or temporary erectile dysfunction is a definite unhealthy body clue. And in all cases, if you feel that you're over-training, there's only one thing you should do: rest! Take some time off. Just as your muscles need rest after a strenuous workout, your penis needs rest too. Depending on how much you over-trained, the impotence rarely lasts more than a few days.

Along with giving your penis rest, you may also want to use warm ups and gentle massages to help improve blood flow. In Appendix A, you'll also find a list of vitamins that increase hardness and penile blood flow under the section "Penis Supplements."

There are two things you shouldn't do in the midst of temporary erectile dysfunction. First, don't dwell on the problem. When you get anxious and nervous, your body pumps out adrenalin quicker than a bartender at Mardi Gras pumps out Bud Light—and adrenalin is the kryptonite of your erections. It's ironic, but the more you think about not having an erection, the harder time you will have maintaining one. The second thing you should avoid, at least until your erections return to normal, is sex and masturbation. This is important, as putting any type of stress on your penis will only aggravate the problem. Give your penis the time it needs to heal.

Also keep in mind that the erectile dysfunction might not even be caused by performing penis exercises—and therefore could not be temporary. Stress, unhealthy eating habits, lack of physical exercise, unbalanced hormones, and a variety of other problems all lead to erectile dysfunction. See a doctor if your hardness troubles last longer than a week.

His Story

Over-training

Andrew was frightened. He was only 30 years old, and everything was fine just a day ago. Andrew decided to increase the intensity three-fold and jelq for an entire hour, despite the fact he had only been performing penis exercises for three weeks. "I was hoping I could gain even quicker," he later told me.

The outcome wasn't what he was hoping for. Andrew hadn't been able to achieve an erection in the last twenty-four hours—since his last workout. Andrew asked for my help with the community help service at http://www.PEGym.com.

I gave Andrew the basic recommendations: stop all penis exercises, avoid sex and masturbation, gently massage the penis, and apply frequent warm ups throughout the day to help the healing process. I also informed Andrew that no matter how soon he recovered, even if by the next day he was experiencing normal erections again, he should still give his penis rest. Exercising too soon will only beget more problems.

I also told Andrew to put his negative thoughts aside (he was already contemplating how bad life would be without his "best friend"). Even though over-training and poor erection quality shouldn't be taken lightly, it's almost always temporary and shouldn't send the mind speeding quicker than Jeff Gordon on race day. The best thing anyone can do in the instance of over-training is relax. I suggested to Andrew that he probably just went overboard and now has to sit on the bench for a few days.

Andrew followed my advice, and emailed me again two days later. He reported that his situation was better, but his penis remained floppy and spongy. "There's inflation, but no hardness," he said. Andrew also told me he went to see a doctor. "The doctor," Andrew told me, "confirmed that the penis is very pliable, and he doesn't believe there will be any long-term damage."

Andrew made a good decision by seeking medical help. Some men avoid the doctor at all costs, simply because they are embarrassed. Talking to the doctor about sexual issues, and especially about penis exercises, is indeed an awkward conversation, but it might be a necessary one.

I then reinforced the idea that Andrew was recovering. He was showing great progress thus far, so it would make sense for him to keep following the advice I gave him.

And he did. Three days later, Andrew declared, "I'm now off the bench, warming up, and ready to bat!"

"What's the Worst That Could Happen?"

In my experience with penis exercises and talking to thousands of penis exercisers, nearly every scary incident has ended similar to Andrew's—frightening, yet quickly back to normal. Nevertheless, similar to how several people have gone beyond their limits in a sport and caused a sprain, a few men have gone beyond their limits in performing penis exercises and caused temporary erectile dysfunction—for several months on a few very rare occasions.

Severe over-training, in which temporary erectile dysfunction or another serious problem occurred for more than a week, is rare. In fact, you're probably more likely to cause serious harm to your penis during intense sex or masturbation than with penis exercises. But keep in mind that you can cause long-term harm to your penis if you use more intensity than you can handle. Many of the recommendations in this book are based on the fact that your penis health always comes first. That's why erect jelqing and stretching are never advised, and why I recommend using light intensity in the beginning.

The bottom line: proceed with caution when performing penis exercises. Your penis isn't "Robocock," despite what your partner tells you. If at any time you feel something is wrong, it probably is. Don't use an exercise unless you're sure your penis can handle it. In the long run, this will mean saving time, seeing results, and avoiding any over-training injuries. The good news is that the body has a magnificent ability to take care of itself. The penis is a durable organ and it tends to quickly overcome anything that is thrown at it. Naturally, your body goes to great lengths to protect the organ that leads to your offspring.

34

The End of the First 5 Weeks

For most men, the first five weeks is a mixed bag. Your first gains will probably be accompanied by feelings of doubt, astonishment, and wonder—often a wonder about why you didn't know about performing penis exercises sooner. Several men make great gains during this beginning period. On the other hand, some men don't gain a thing.

Question: "I haven't gained at all during the first five weeks. What should I do?"

The most important thing you can do is persist and not give up. Make sure your mindset is right. Penis exercising is about more than just adding size; it's about having a healthy and hard penis as well. The men who usually don't gain are the ones who are so eager that they rush the entire process and in turn set themselves up for failure.

Keep in mind that numerous men don't gain for several months and then all of a sudden—seemingly out of the blue—they gain. If you didn't gain, there's a reason. Make sure you are following all the tips in Chapter 31: Maximizing Gains. Additionally, use your body clues to help you find out the problem.

If you have hard erections and healthy body clues, then perhaps the Basic Beginner's Routine wasn't intense enough for you. Healthy body clues are good news, because in this next part of the book, I will go over key ways to intensify your routine.

On the other hand, perhaps the Basic Beginner's Routine was too intense, which is especially evident if you experienced unhealthy body clues. If so, take a week or more off and come back with a much lighter routine, such as one of the routines in Chapter 28.

Did You Reach Your Goal?

After you hit your goal, you'll need to follow a cementing routine, lasting roughly three months. A cementing routine will help "cement" your gains in an effort to make them permanent. After your growth is cemented, your normal everyday erections—combined with a light maintenance routine—will typically provide enough exercise to maintain your new penis size. If you reached your goal, skip to Chapter 41: Cementing Your Goal.

Are You Ready to Advance?

You most likely still have a ways to go. Part V will go over ways to advance your routine. But before you move forth, ask yourself the following questions: Do you have healthy body clues? Most importantly, are you ready to advance? That is, do you feel comfortable increasing the intensity?

If so, you're ready to move on .

Part IV Review

- ✓ The Basic Beginner's Routine is a general guideline. The best thing you can do is pay attention to your body clues and move up accordingly.
- ✓ Every man's penis is different genetically and physically, and this causes problems with "set" routines.
- ✓ There is no set limit on how much—or how little—you exercise. If you can gain with less intensity, go for it.
- ✓ Depending on your unique goals, choose the exercises that best suit you.
- ✓ Common side effects include the darkening effect, the doughnut effect, and spotting along the penis.
- ✓ Uncommon side effects include the appearance of bruises, blisters, and blood.
- ✓ Temporary erectile dysfunction, when in correspondence with performing penis exercises, is most often caused by over-training

Important Pages from Part IV:

- ➢ Basic Beginner's Routine, page 98
- ➢ Progressive Routine, page 100
- ➢ Least Work/Max Gain Routine, page 104
- ➢ Ways to Maximize Gains, page 116
- ➢ Overcoming Possible Side Effects, page 122

After the First 5 Weeks

Part V

In this part you will:

- Adopt an advanced routine, which you will use beyond the first five weeks
- Learn how to increase the intensity using advanced exercises and other methods
- Discover key ways to maximize your gains as you advance
- Learn how a long break helps reignite your gains
- Find a cementing routine to use once you reach your goal

35

Advancing

"Every day it will get longer and longer. I promise you it will grow. It will eventually get longer, I promise you."

– *Arnold Schwarzenegger, telling Conan O'Brien how to enlarge his penis*

Penis exercising is a journey. And like most journeys, it has its ups and its downs. Also similar to most journeys, the end result is what makes the whole trip worth it. You finished the first part of your journey. These next few chapters will guide you on what to do as you advance the rest of the way. You won't be changing much. Just adding advanced exercises and a few more guidelines.

The Advancing Guidelines

Ideally, you will continually gain and reach your goal fairly quickly. But, as with all ideal circumstances this doesn't always happen. In fact, many men find that as they advance, they hit a plateau—in which the gains slow down and eventually hit a big red stop-sign. Some men experience a plateau fairly quickly, just after a month or two. Other men never hit a plateau.

You can maximize your growth and decrease your chances of reaching a plateau by following three simple guidelines (and even if you do hit a plateau, there are a couple of ways to overcome it, which you will learn about later).

Guideline 1 - Always jelq:

As you advance, you'll learn several advanced exercises. But regardless of how many advanced exercises you use, you should still always jelq. Think of this exercise as your star quarterback—it plays a vital role to any penis exercises routine and shouldn't be put on the sidelines. The jelq is the best exercise for moving blood throughout the penis and is a great intermission between girth and length exercises.

Guideline 2 - Change it up:

As you know, your body has a remarkable ability to adapt. Similar to your muscles, your penis needs to be constantly challenged for it to grow. The easiest way to keep the penis off guard, and therefore make it harder to adapt, is to switch up the exercises used often. Every few weeks, try to change your workout as much as possible. Change the exercises you use, the number of reps you do for each exercise, and even the order in which you do the exercises. Changing the exercises you use will be easier to do after a few more months, when you have plenty of different exercises to choose from. As time goes on, you may even want to switch up the number of days you perform penis exercises each week. In Chapter 38, there are several effective advanced routines. Each of them provides a great way to add variety to your workouts. As time goes on, mix it up and try each of them.

The goal is to keep your penis off guard. As one man says, "Irregularity is the number one principle I have followed to make big penis enlargement gains. I've gained over three inches and I attribute most of my gains to penis exercises as sporadically as possible. I change my entire routine in any way I can. One week, for example, I'll perform penis exercises for three days, and then take four days off. The next week I 'll do it one on, one off. The next: five on, two off. The bottom line: I constantly keep my penis guessing."

Guideline 3 - Continue to increase the intensity and watch your body clues:

Always focus on these principles. Particularly, continue to increase the intensity (unless you have unhealthy body clues, of course!). Too many times I've seen penis exercisers slow down after the beginner's routine, only to see their gains dramatically slow down too.

Similar to your body, as your penis becomes conditioned to the exercises, growth will slow to a halt unless your penis is pushed beyond what it is use to. Hollywood fitness guru Gunnar Peterson warns in his book, The Workout, "Your body learns to adapt quickly to constant stress. Keep repeating 'any' exercise or activity and your body eventually wises up." The rate at which growth occurs often slows down a bit after the initial five weeks (as with all exercising, the first few steps are often the most beneficial); but by repeatedly exercising your penis beyond what it is accustomed to, you'll continually make the most of your gains.

In the beginning stage, you increased the intensity in one major way: by exercising for longer periods. As you transition into the advanced stage, you'll have two other ways to increase the intensity of your exercises. The first way is to add advanced exercises into the mix. Although you don't need to use every advanced exercise, they do enable you to add variety. By the end of six months, you'll have over 40 different exercises to choose from. The second way you can increase the intensity is to make the exercises you've already been using even more intense, which can be done in a variety of ways. For instance, you can kegel while jelqing and stretching. Over the next couple of chapters, I will go over these two important aspects of increasing the intensity in more detail.

36

Advanced Exercises

Three men walk out of a bar and stop on a small bridge to empty their bladders. They lean out over the edge in the dark and begin to urinate. The first man says, "River sure is cold."

The second man says, "It's deep, too."

The third man says, "Sandy bottom."

Thus far, you've only used a couple of basic exercises. As you advance, your choices will greatly expand. Advanced exercises have helped many men reach their goal. They have helped hard gainers gain and easy gainers gain faster. That's because by using various exercises, and by changing them up as often as possible, you aren't consistently using the same formula (just jelqs, stretches, and kegels). This variety makes it harder for your penis to adapt and hit a plateau.

The Different Advanced Exercises

The advanced exercises are largely broken down into two categories: length and girth (with the exception of the three advanced kegel exercises). The advanced length exercises focus on stretching, whereas the girth exercises largely focus on expanding the penis. The best expansion exercises work by stopping blood from leaving the penis, causing it to go the only way it can: outward. Because you get the most expansion when the penis is erect, many of the advanced girth exercises are done when you have an erection. There is more of a risk when you do erect exercises, so don't take them lightly.

The best part about the advanced exercises is that you can mix them and match them, change them around during each workout, and use those that feel most comfortable to you. All you have to do is avoid exercising too intense too soon.

Intensity Levels

Some exercises are more intense than others. A few of the advanced exercises can be added to your routine right away; some exercises can't be used for at least six months. To help you determine how intense each exercise is, I've broken the exercises down into intensity levels. The intensity levels range from one to five (one being the least intense, and five being the most intense).

Intensity Level 1:

Includes the basic exercises you've already been doing (the kegel, the jelq, and the basic stretch).

Intensity Level 2:

The start of the advanced exercises. Level 2 exercises include three new kegel exercises, two new stretches (or length exercises), and two girth exercises. You can start using these right away, or whenever you feel comfortable doing so.

Intensity Level 3:

Includes more stretches along with two jelq variations, which are effective in obtaining girth and fixing a penis curve. Avoid using these exercises until you have been consistently performing penis exercises for at least two to three months total. Meaning, you've only been performing penis exercises for a total of one month if you exercised your penis for three weeks, took three months off, and then exercised for another week. In this instance, you'll need to perform penis exercise for an additional one to two months before you can use these exercises.

Intensity Level 4:

The start of erect girth exercises. If you choose to do exercises while erect, use caution and pay close attention to your body clues. Level 4 also includes more intense stretches. Avoid using these exercises until you have been consistently performing penis exercises for three to four months total.

Intensity Level 5:

Includes several more girth exercises that are done while erect, along with an additional intense stretch. Avoid using these exercises until you have been performing penis exercises for four to six months total.

All of the advanced exercises and their Intensity Levels are located in Appendix C. Also in Appendix C is the Exercise Guide, which has a "Recommended Number of Months Before Use" column for each exercise. Avoid using a certain exercise before its recommended time. The recommended time slot doesn't fit everyone's individual needs. Some men need more time; others need less. Nevertheless, you'll over-train if you use an advance exercise before your penis is ready, and this will lead to temporary erectile dysfunction and possibly something even worse. The best way to optimize gains and minimize over-training injuries is to avoid jumping into the advanced exercises before the recommendation. Also, when you start using a new exercise, use it lightly.

Advanced Exercises Aren't Necessary

Just because an exercise is advanced doesn't necessarily mean you will advance your gains by using it, especially if you use it at the wrong time. You don't have to use all of the advanced exercises. In fact, you don't have to use any of them. Several men have gained multiple inches just by jelqing and stretching. You most likely can too, so long as you make sure to increase the intensity in the other ways.

You might, however, have specific goals that can't be met without using advanced exercises. A good example of this is if your goal is to gain girth, but you find yourself gaining mainly length, then you will most likely have to add some advanced girth exercises to your routine if you want to reach your goal. Regardless, there might be a number of exercises you will not like. That's okay. Skip those exercises. With over thirty different exercises to choose from, you have plenty of choices. And if you sign online, there are even more choices. Men are constantly discovering new exercises, and you can always check out http://www.PEGym.com/penis-exercises to learn about them.

You should only add new exercises when you feel comfortable with the exercises that you are currently using. The goal is to try to become in tune with your penis, its wants, and its needs. The best way to do this is to let your measurements and your body clues guide you.

37

Increasing the Intensity of Your Exercises

You can increase the intensity of the exercises you've already been using by slightly changing various aspects of each exercise. Keep in mind you'll want to incorporate the following options gradually—not all at once.

Increase the amount of time you spend on each rep:

As a rule, the longer the rep lasts—whether it's each stretch, squeeze, or jelq stroke—the more intense the exercise is. For example, the typical jelq lasts two to three seconds. If you make the jelq stroke slower, lasting five seconds or more, you'll increase the entire jelqing effect. To get the most out of your jelqs, work up to slow 10-second jelq strokes.

Another example is to hold your stretches for longer periods. In the beginning, you held each stretch for roughly 30 seconds. As you advance, hold the stretch for as long as you feel comfortable—up to one, three, and even five minutes or more.

Increase the pressure and force used:

Increasing the amount of force you use to grip, stretch, and jelq the penis is a surefire way to increase the intensity.

Increase your erection level:

The more engorged your penis, the more intense the exercise. As time goes on, you can start jelqing and stretching with higher erection levels (but keep in mind that jelqing at higher erection levels targets girth and jelqing at lower erection levels targets length).

Add kegels:

Kegeling while doing other penis exercises often intensifies the entire workout—especially when stretching upward. That's because kegeling contracts the pelvic floor muscles at the base of the inner penis. As a result, the kegel adds more leverage to the stretch. Think of it as your penis being pulled in two different directions (in one direction by your hand; in the other direction by your pelvic floor muscles). Just as useful, kegeling while doing girth exercises pushes more blood into the penis, which causes more engorgement.

Use multiple angles:

Stretch, jelq, and squeeze in every angle possible. Most important, stretch any way achievable. Stretch up, down, left, right, left-down, right-up, etc. Using multiple angles is important because different angles target different areas of the penis, and thus maximizes your potential for growth. For instance, stretching up targets the inner penis and stretching down targets the ligaments. But don't just diversify your stretches. Do every exercise in multiple angles. Jelq up, down, left, and right. Keep it as varied as possible.

Flex your abs:

Flexing your abs while stretching your penis increases the power of the stretch. Flexing is especially useful when stretching downward. That's because the fundiform ligament—which encircles the base of the penis—connects the abs to the penis. Similar to kegeling while stretching, flexing your abs while stretching pulls your penis in two directions.

Add a device:

For the first three to six months, you'll want to stick to using just your hands and, at most, a penis extender. But as your penis becomes more conditioned, you might consider using a device to help intensify your routine. Many men report that using a device helps. In fact, some men use only devices. In Appendix A under the section "Penis Enlargement Devices," you'll find more information on devices.

38

Basic Advancing Routine

This chapter lays out the Basic Advancing Routine. It continues where the Basic Beginner's Routine left off.

The Basic Advancing Routine

Four days a week, do the following:

The main workout:

- 5 minute warm up
- 10 minutes of length (stretching)
- 20 minutes of jelqing
- 5 minutes of girth

Anytime throughout the workout day:

- 100 JAI stretches
- 5 minutes of kegel exercises

Everyday:

- Do the kegel start/stop every time you use the restroom.

Four days a week, for now:

Increase to five days a week when you feel that you and your penis are ready. Overtime, your penis will need less rest as it becomes more conditioned to the exercises.

Increase the Intensity:

Continue to increase the intensity in accordance with your body clues and your gains. Do this by adding more time, adding more exercises, and increasing the intensity of the exercises you are using.

Warm Up:

Continue to do a ten minute warm up if you want, but five minutes will typically suffice after the first five weeks. Just make sure it's thorough.

Length:

You now have three stretches to choose from: the basic stretch, the pendulum stretch, and the rotating stretch (the last two are found in the Exercise Guide in Appendix C). Change it up and keep it varied. As time goes on, continue to add more length exercises according to the recommendation found in the Exercise Guide.

Jelqing:

By the end of your second month, you can start incorporating the jelq variations: the vertical jelq and the side jelq. But for now, gradually increase the intensity of your jelqs by using more force, jelqing at multiple angles, and making your jelq strokes last longer.

Girth:

For the next two months you have two girth exercises to work with. Gradually add more girth exercises according to the recommendation found in the Exercise Guide (Appendix C). Eventually, you 'll be able to use all ten girth exercises.

Kegels:

For now, kegel five minutes a day, four times a week. You can use any kegel exercise, including the advanced kegel exercises located in Appendix C. As you advance, you can try increasing to ten minutes per workout day. Most men, however, find that five minutes of kegeling four to five days a week is plenty of exercise to keep their pelvic floor muscles in good shape.

39

Alternative Advancing Routines

Question: "I'm looking for a more specific advanced routine. Can you help me out?"

Finding a "perfect" advanced routine is complicated. In many instances it's even impossible. Recall that everyone is different. So what works for you won't necessarily work for the guy down the block, and vice versa.

Let me give you an example that involves an unfortunately common theme in the penis exercises community. When a man makes big gains or reaches his goal, he often lets the community know what routine and exercises helped him—typically by posting them online via a penis exercises forum. This is great, as it adds to the collective knowledge of the penis exercises world. But more often than not, the exercises and routines are both advanced, and this is where many men get off track.

Understandably, several men believe that since the advanced routine worked for the other guy, it will probably work for them. So, what do they do? They completely duplicate the routine, without personalizing it to their body's wants and needs. I've seen this happen time after time.

The guy who is doing the copying often jumps into this completely different—and typically much more advanced—routine.

After all is said and done, the man who jumps into the new routine is usually left disappointed. He might experience a small spurt of growth, but this growth is often nowhere near what the original guy reported and is typically followed by a plateau or, in worst cases, an over-training injury —none of which is productive.

The reason that the routine worked for the other guy is simple. The actual advanced routine isn't what produced the growth. It's how the man's penis reacted to the routine. That's why it's important to follow the guidelines (always jelq, change it up, watch your body clues closely, gradually increase the intensity, and get enough rest). These principles guide your routine more than any set number of jelq, stretches, and kegels ever could.

That said, if you're looking for ways to add variety to your routine as you advance, the possibilities really are limitless. Over the next few pages, there are five popular advanced routines and workouts that have helped many men reach their goal. You can find more routines at http://www.PEGym.com/routines.

As you advance, use them as a general guideline to help you change it up and keep your penis from getting too comfortable to the exercises. Depending on how much time you typically spend on a workout, the amount of time listed on each routine is variable. For example, if you're up to performing penis exercises fifty minutes per workout, you won't want to cut back to only exercising twenty minutes. Instead, adapt the following routines to your current workout plan. This goes for all the example routines listed in this chapter. Also continue to do your JAI Stretches and kegels according to the Basic Advancing Routine's recommendation.

Alternative Routine 1: The Progressive Routine

Similar to the Beginner's Progressive Routine, this routine adds a certain amount of jelqs, length exercises, and girth exercises each week.

The Advanced Progressive Routine

Four days a week, do the following:

The main workout:

- 5 minute warm up
- 12 minutes of length
- 12 minutes of jelqing
- 5 minutes of girth

Increasing the intensity:

Each week add:

- 1 minute of jelqing
- 1 minute of length
- 1 minute of girth

Alternative Routine 2: The Least Work/Max Gain Routine

If you gained with the Beginner's Least Work/Max Gain Routine, try this advanced variation.

The Advanced Least Work/Max Gain Routine

Do the workout, and then rest for 2 days. Do this for a total of 6 workouts (18 total days). Thereafter, do light exercises for 1 week. Then take 1 month off.

The main workout:

- 5 minute warm up
- 15 minutes of length
- 25 minutes of jelqing
- 10 minutes of girth

1 week of light exercising:

For seven days, do the following every day:

- 5 minutes of length
- 5 minutes of girth
- 5 minutes of jelqing

1 month break:

During the month-long break, don't do any exercises that actually exercise your penis, such as the jelq. Continue to kegel.

Repeat:

After the break, repeat the 6 workout days, the 1 week cementing stage, and the 1 month break as many times as you can gain doing so. But each time around, add more time and exercises to the routine.

Alternative Routine 3: The Split Routine

This routine splits your workout into two smaller workouts: one in the morning, one in the evening.

The Split Routine

Four days a week, do the following:

Morning workout:

- 5 minute warm up
- 15 minutes of jelqing
- 10 minutes of girth

Evening workout:

- 5 minute warm up
- 20 minutes of length

Alternative Routine 4: The Alternate Routine

With this routine, you alternate the days you work out.

The Alternate Routine

Repeat this cycle:

- Workout one day, rest two days
- Workout two days, rest three days
- Workout three days, rest four days
- Workout four days, rest three days
- Workout five days, rest two days
- Workout six days, rest for a week.
- Repeat

The main workout:

- 5 minute warm up
- 15 minutes of length
- 15 minutes of jelqing
- 15 minutes of girth

Alternative Routine 5: Plateau-Breaking "Shock Workout"

This intense kind of workout has helped many men break a plateau. The idea of this routine is to "shock" your penis into gaining by using much more intensity than you've been using, yet at the same time not go overboard. Because of its intensity, a shock workout isn't recommended unless you've been performing penis exercises for several months. Also, you'll need to give your penis multiple days of rest after a shock workout.

How often you use this workout is up to you. Some men do a shock workout every once in a blue moon to help kick-start their gains, whereas other men consistently do nothing but shock workouts once or twice a week.

The Plateau-Breaking "Shock Workout"

A typical shock workout lasts anywhere from two to four times longer than your normal workout—depending on how long you've been performing penis exercises. The longer you've been performing penis exercises, the more extra time your penis will be able to handle.

For your first shock workout:

- Give your penis two to three days of complete rest from penis exercises prior to the workout.
- For the actual workout, do double your normal workout. For example, if you normally workout for 45 minutes, then try a 90 minute workout.
- After the workout, give your penis at least three to six days of rest.

For future shock workouts:

If you experienced healthy body clues a few days after your first shock workout, try increasing the intensity. Gradually try three, four, and even five times your normal workout. Some penis exercisers eventually work up to eight to twelve-hour shock workouts (split up throughout the day and generally with the help of a device so they can focus their time on other things). Either way, for the best results, always give your penis plenty of rest prior to and after the shock workout.

40

Plateaus and Breaks

As you venture forth through weeks, months, or even years of performing penis exercises, hopefully you will be showered with consistent gains. But at some point, the gains may slow down and possibly even stop all together. After all, you're not likely to end up with a 24" penis that is 12" in girth. Your body simply can't produce such a thing. In any case, such size would be counterproductive, as few, if any, women would want to play with you.

If you ever get to this uneventful point—in which you've tried it all but it just isn't working anymore—stop performing penis exercises. Quit. Layoff. Take a vacation. Whatever you do, don't continue what you've been doing. If it didn't work today, it most likely won't work tomorrow, either.

Why would this happen? In simple terms, your penis is just following the natural laws of biology—it's adapting to the exercises. Think of it as your penis seeing the exercises as a threat. So it builds a shield against the exercises. As time goes on, you will have to use more and more exercises to penetrate the shield—and gain even more. You may eventually get to a point in which nothing penetrates the shield. Your penis stops growing and an unwanted plateau shows up.

Over the years, the men of the penis exercises community have learned that one of the best ways to overcome a plateau is to take a break. That's because during a break, the penis eventually lowers its shield. So when you return, you will be able to gain.

Several penis exercisers have confessed that their most prominent gains were also their early gains. Fortunately, many men find that after they take an extended *"deconditioning"* break, their penis is often as receptive to the exercises as when they first started performing penis exercises.

Depending on the conditioned state of your penis (that is, how adapted your penis is to the exercises and how long you've been exercising) an effective break lasts six to twelve weeks. Many men find that two months is an optimal amount of time to renew growth.

Since you're not cementing your gains when you break, some of your gains might be temporarily lost. It's even possible that you'll lose all of your gains. This is uncommon, but it happens. The permanency of your gains largely depends on how long ago you made the gains. Generally speaking, any gains you made three or more months ago are probably permanent. Either way, don't worry. Gains are easier to recapture the second time around. Most men find that they restore their gains and even add more to their size within just a few weeks of returning.

When you come back from a break, you'll want to start out lighter than what you left with. Your penis won't be as strong, or as conditioned, so less exercise will often do the trick. Depending on the length of the break, you may find that when you return you can even gain with a beginning routine. Moreover, since your penis is less conditioned than it was before, starting out where you left off will most likely lead to over-training The best thing you can do is start out light and rapidly work your way back to where you left off.

You can still kegel while on break. So if you hate sitting around while you can be actively improving, try spending the extended break focusing on your kegels. Pull a Tiger Woods on your pelvic floor muscles: really get in there and perfect your kegel routine.

If a long break doesn't sound appealing, but you really can't get past a plateau, then try taking several little breaks. Go for one week on, one week off. You may also want to look into penis enlargement devices, which have helped many men. For more information on devices, see the "Penis Enlargement Devices" section in Appendix A. Another thing you might want to try is the Plateau-Breaking "Shock Routine" (outlined in the previous chapter).

His Story

What a break did for me

When Chris hit a plateau after roughly five months of performing penis exercises, he was stuck between a rock and a hard place. He was only half-way to his goal, but committed to not giving up. In an effort to jump start his gains, Chris did what many others do: he tried using a penis enlargement device—such as a hanger or an extender. Chris went for hanging. Although many men make extravagant gains with devices, Chris did not. He eventually worked his way up to hanging several hours each week, but the ruler measurements kept coming back with the same numbers.

After nearly a year of ample work and no growth, Chris realized, "If I haven't gained yet, something must be wrong." Still committed to reaching his goal, Chris did some research. He heard that taking an extended break will possibly restart his growth, so he took three months off from performing penis exercises.

When Chris came back, he was surprised to find that his gains rolled in rapidly. He nearly gained as much as he did when he first started performing penis exercises. Even better, Chris declared, "Taking a break not only gave my penis a rest, but it gave my mind a rest too. The exercises gradually became more boring and tiresome than anything." He eventually understood that these breaks were needed to keep his mind fresh, and his motivation high.

To stop himself from hitting another plateau, Chris set himself on a strict penis exercises routine, cycling between exercising and breaks —

exercising for six weeks, and breaking for twelve weeks. Chris finally reached his goal after five cycles, and says, "I'm finally happy with my nine-inch penis."

Interval Training

Until recently, men were often advised to perform penis exercises through a plateau—often unsuccessfully. "Do whatever it takes," was the mantra. Fortunately, the discovery of the deconditioning break showed that one of the easiest ways to keep gains coming isn't to work through a plateau; it's to work around it using the same method that Chris used: rotate between taking a break and exercising.

This kind of training is termed interval training, which can be done in one of two ways. The first way—and often the easiest—is to just penis exercise until you reach a plateau (if you ever do), and then take a two or three month break. This is the best option for now, as there is no telling if you'll ever hit a plateau. Several men just keep on gaining, never having to worry about plateaus or breaks. If you later find that you're susceptible to plateaus, try the second way—do what Chris did: set yourself on a plan in which you exercise for three or four weeks, then break for six or more weeks.

41

Cementing Your Goal

You've made the gains. Now you want to keep them. To do this, you'll have to follow a cementing routine and possibly do a light penile workout on occasion; this is known as maintenance.

Maintenance

Nothing in life lasts forever. From the style of clothes you wear to the cells in your body, everything has an expiration date. The same goes for penis size. As you know, your penis will eventually grow old—and this often leads to shrinking and contracting. So, in this regard, your gains are never permanent. Aging is a fact of life.

But because you've been blessed with the knowledge of penis exercises, you are equipped to combat the attacks of aging. By periodically performing penis exercises here and there, you can make your new-found penis size last a lifetime. Maintenance also has another benefit: it helps keep your penis hard and healthy throughout the rest of your life. When most men reach an age in which they turn to drugs like Viagra, a man with a well maintained penis won't have to.

Compared to what you've been using, a maintenance workout is a light and simple workout. Most maintenance routines consist of either doing two to three minutes of jelqs and stretches every day or so, or doing a light penis exercises workout once or twice a week. One penis exerciser recounts his maintenance routine: "Every time I take a shower, I do twenty to thirty jelqs and two to three minutes of stretching. I also do several kegels throughout the day. I look at these exercises as a daily task that must be done, such as brushing my teeth. This light 'shower maintenance' has allowed me to keep my gains for years and even added a little more to my size."

A maintenance routine, however, isn't necessarily required to keep the penis enlargement gains you've made. Some men quit performing penis exercises over ten years ago and haven't lost a millimeter. These men successfully cemented their gains. As one penis exerciser who uses the online alias Memento put it, "I stopped performing penis exercises ages ago. I lost a bit after I stopped but since then my gains have been stable and I do no maintenance exercises."

Other men haven't been as lucky, especially the men who had to stop performing penis exercises abruptly because of severe over-training When a man severely over-trains, he often loses a big chunk of his gains, largely because it knocks cementing out of the question (when you over-train, you have to stop performing penis exercises). Additionally, going extremely overboard can lead to poor erection quality for several weeks or more; and weak erections put a damper on sex and everyday erections, which are other methods for maintaining penile growth.

Obtain Frequent Erections

A chief reason the gains from performing penis exercises are permanent is most likely because of the primary purpose of the penis: to obtain adequate erections. Because erections are a light form of penis exercise, everyday sexual activity sometimes provides enough of a workout to keep the penis in its new size. The more erections you have, and the longer you sustain these erections, the more likely your gains will be permanent.

Generally, length gains are easier to cement than girth gains and whatever you gained three or more months ago is usually yours to keep. Some men say their gains are cemented the day they make the gain; other men say they need to perform penis exercises for at least three additional months after they make a gain before it is permanent. To play it safe, you'll want to follow a cementing routine.

Cementing

You can cement your growth in two ways. The first way is to overshoot your goal. That is, if your goal is to have an eight-inch penis, continue exercising until you reach eight-and-a-half inches. Going beyond your goal is the most sensible way to cement your growth, as over time many men often lose the last quarter inch or so they gained.

The second way, and the most common, is to gradually decrease the intensity over three to four months. For instance, once you've reached your goal, continue performing penis exercises with the same routine for a month, then cut the amount of time spent performing penis exercises in half. A month later, again cut the routine in half, and so on.

You May Need to Cement More than Once

Even if you follow a cementing routine, all of your growth might not completely cement the first time around. You may lose a few millimeters. You may lose even more. Either way, don't panic. Just like skeletal muscles, the penis seemingly has a "memory" of its largest size, as growth is almost always easier to recapture the second time around. Whenever you start performing penis exercises again, your lost gains will most likely return fairly quickly.

You can avoid having to "recapture" your lost gains by tracking your measurements closely as you start the cementing phase. If your gains start slipping, then wean yourself off your routine at a slower pace.

Example Cementing Routine

Here is an example cementing routine. Your personal cementing needs will vary. The more time you spend cementing, the greater chance your gains will be permanent.

Before the cementing routine:

- As some loss of growth often occurs, overshoot your goal by a quarter inch in length, girth, or both. Gaining beyond your goal will increase your chances of keeping your desired penis size. After you reach your overshot goal, continue to the first month of the cementing routine.

Month 1:

- Continue using the routine that you acquired your most recent gains with.

Month 2:

- Use half the routine that you acquired your most recent gains with. For example, if you reached your overshot goal by performing penis exercises four days a week for sixty minutes each day, then either penis exercise two days a week, sixty minutes each day; or four days a week for thirty minutes each day.

Month 3:

- Use one quarter of your original routine.

After the cementing routine:

- Perform some penile maintenance every now and then. For example, do a few minutes of penis exercises each day while in the shower. Also, to keep your penis healthy and hard, continue to do kegels and the kegel start/stop.

Part V Review

- ✓ As you advance: always jelq, continue to watch your body clues, and change it up frequently in an effort to "keep your penis guessing."
- ✓ Continue to increase the intensity. You now have three ways to do this: add more time, intensify the exercises you've been using, and add advance exercises.
- ✓ All of the exercises are broken down into 'Intensity Levels.' Avoid using any exercise before its "recommended time," which is found in the Exercise Guide in Appendix C.
- ✓ Advanced exercises aren't necessary. Moreover, just because an exercise is advanced, doesn't mean you will advance in gains using it, especially if your penis isn't ready.
- ✓ If you ever get to the point in which you've tried it all but it just isn't working anymore, take a six to twelve week break from performing penis exercises. Many men find that this renews their growth.
- ✓ To make your gains permanent, you'll have to follow a cementing routine, which involves weaning yourself off performing penis exercises over three months time.

Important Pages from Part V:

- ➢ The Advancing Guidelines, page 144
- ➢ Breakdown of the Intensity Levels, page 148
- ➢ The Basic Advancing Routine, page 154
- ➢ Alternative Routines, page 157
- ➢ Example Cementing Routine, 172

Appendix A:

Eleven Questions Men Ask Relating to Penis Exercising

In this part we will discuss:

- Question #1 - Time is Limited
- Question #2 - Fixing a Penis Curve
- Question #3 - Becoming Multi-Orgasmic
- Question #4 - Erection Difficulties
- Question #5 - Penis Supplements
- Question #6 -Penis Enlargement Pills
- Question #7 - Gaining Troubles
- Question #8 - Penis Enlargement Devices
- Question #9 - Penis Enlargement Survey
- Question #10 - Increasing Flaccid Size
- Question #11 - Premature Ejaculation

1. Time is Limited

Question: "I don't have a lot of time. Can I still build a bigger, harder and healthier penis?"

Answer: Absolutely. If your time is limited, the first place to start is the Least Work/Max Gain Routine. With this light routine, you'll only perform penis exercises six days a month, and only twelve minutes each day. After you've been using the Least Work/Max Gain Routine for a while, you can move up to the advanced version.

Another great way you can maximize your time is to follow the old African proverb that asks the question, "How do you eat an elephant?" The answer: "One bite at a time." The take home message: Things are much easier to accomplish when they are broken into pieces. You can save time by breaking your routine into portions throughout the day. Do your jelqs, for example, in the morning and your other exercises at night. Or even break your routine into three, four, and even five mini sessions—whatever works for you. In the worst case scenario, you can do one to three minutes of penis exercises each time you go to the bathroom and then do another five to ten minutes when you take a shower. This way, you're not blocking out huge chunks of your day, yet you are still putting in the effort—no matter how busy you are.

Numerous penis exercisers report that they got their best results when they split their routine into smaller workouts. That's because after thirty to forty minutes of performing penis exercises, the whole thing can seem more like a tedious job and less like a fun, productive hobby. Towards the end of a long workout, several men find that they start doing their exercises with half the effort; and half the effort leads to half the results. When the workouts are kept short, it often makes them more fun, lively, and effective.

Another thing you can do is circuit your exercises. Go straight from one exercise to the next, without ever taking a break. Not giving your penis any rest between exercises provides an intense workout in less time. Circuits are particularly useful when you get into the later Intensity Levels and have plenty of exercises to choose from. A few example circuit exercises are located in Appendix C. Try them out after you feel comfortable doing Intensity Level 5 exercises.

If time becomes a big problem, by all means take a break. You can always come back when you have more time and more motivation. In fact, many men find that the best way to perform penis exercise is to do it in spurts—do it for several weeks, make some gains, take a break, and repeat.

Lastly, as you advance, you may want to consider using a penis enlargement device. Several devices don't take any work at all. You plop on the device and you're good to go quicker than a Crunchwrap Supreme from Taco Bell. For more information, see the "Penis Enlargement Devices" section in this Appendix.

2. Fixing a Penis Curve

Question: "Is a penis curve normal? What causes a curve? Can performing penis exercises fix a curve?"

Answer: A curved penis is nothing to lose sleep over. In fact, a penis curve is fairly normal. "A third of men (33.8 %) have a crooked or curved penis," says Bernice Kanner, author of Are You Normal About Sex, Love, and Relationships?

Moreover, a penis curve often allows the man to stimulate areas that wouldn't otherwise be stimulated. For example, an upward curve provides perfect stimulation to the female G-spot. So it's no surprise that many women love a curved penis. When I was interviewing woman about the most important aspects of a penis, one woman told me, "Nothing gets me off harder than a penis with a curve that hits my spot!" If you have a curve, try using it to your advantage. Get into positions that best suit your curve, and it will most likely best suit your partner too.

"What Causes A Curve?"

A penis curve can be caused by several factors. One cause involves the fact that the main body of the penis is made of three circular chambers, and sometimes one of the three chambers is shorter than the other two—which can be caused by genetics or consistently masturbating with too much pressure on one side of the penis. When one chamber is smaller than the other two, it causes a curve to the shorter side.[1]

It May be Peyronie's Disease

A slight bend in the penis is normal and shouldn't cause too much alarm. But a severe bend that causes physical pain might be Peyronie's disease—plaque formation inside the penis. Peyronie's disease typically has three symptoms:[2]

- *Pain during erection.*
- *A hard lump or tough area where the penis curves.*
- *A curve that forms during adulthood.* "More than 75% of Peyronie's disease patients are between 45 and 65 years old," say the authors of Atlas of Clinical Andrology. If you've had a curve all of your life or the majority of your life, it most likely isn't Peyronie's disease.

Fortunately, Peyronie's disease often heals on its own after twelve to eighteen months, with the curve drastically dissipating. If you experience any pain, or if the curve continues to get worse, see an urologist.

"Can Penis Exercising Fix a Curve?"

Several men have straightened their curve by using certain penis exercises. Some men have even reported that performing penis exercises fixed severe curves, like Peyronie's disease.

The main four exercises for fixing a curve are the straight stretch, the side jelq, the mini jelq, and the straight bend. Depending on the severity of your curve, these four exercises might straighten your penis in as little as one to two months. These curve-fixing exercises are similar to the other exercises throughout this book except they focus on doing the exercise against the curve. If you have a curve that you would like to straighten, use these exercises in place of your normal routine when possible. For example, do the straight stretch in replace of the basic stretch.

Depending on how long you've been performing penis exercises, some of these exercises may be too advanced for you. For instance, you'll want to avoid doing straight bends if you're a beginner. To help you determine when you're ready, use the Exercise Guide in Appendix C, which gives a recommendation on when to use each exercise.

Straight Stretch

The fundamentals of the straight stretch are the same as the basic stretch. But instead of stretching in several different directions, you're only stretching in one direction: opposite of the curve.

If, for instance, your penis curves to the left, then make it your main focus to hold your stretches to the right. Stretching opposite of the curve puts more pressure on the smaller side (in this case the left side), which entices it to grow more. In turn, the smaller side will eventually "catch up" to the bigger side, and the curve will be straightened.

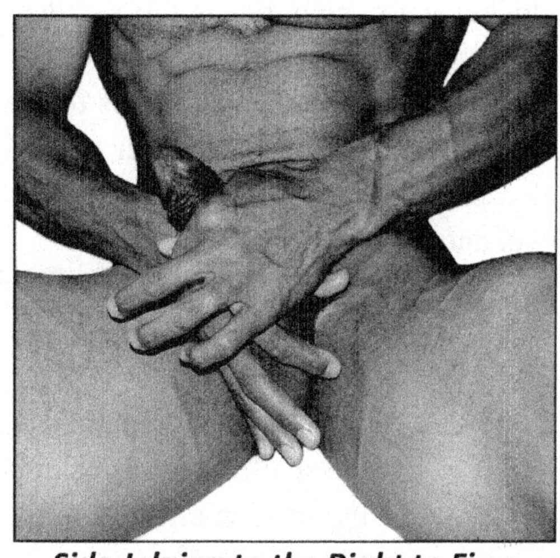

Side Jelqing to the Right to Fix a Left-Hand Curve

The side jelq uses one hand to jelq the penis in the opposite direction of the curve. The other hand encircles the base, which helps stabilize the penis.

Side Jelq

The side jelq is an Intensity Level 3 exercise that jelqs the penis to the left, to the right, back to the left, and so on (see Appendix C for detailed description of how to side jelq).

When your goal is to fix a curve, you'll only side jelq in one direction: against the curve. Again, by placing more pressure on smaller side, you're enticing it to grow more. So if your penis curves to the left, use your left hand to side jelq to the right.

If your penis curves upward, you can use the vertical jelq (described in Appendix C), which focuses bending the penis downwards after each jelq. If it curves downward, do the vertical jelq in reverse (instead of bending downwards, bend upwards.)

Mini Jelq

This exercise will only work if your penis curves either left or right (not up or down). A good understanding of your penis' anatomy will make all the difference in comprehending this exercise, so if you're confused see Appendix B.

The penis consists of three circular chambers. Two top chambers that you see when you look straight down at your penis, and a bottom chamber that holds your urethra. The goal of the mini jelq is to jelq whichever top chamber is the smaller one, and is thus the side the penis curves to. You do this by using a mini pincher grip to focus exclusively on that chamber. If the penis curves to the left, then the left side (the top left corpus chamber) is the smaller side, and thus will be the side you mini jelq. To do the mini jelq, bring your penis to a 50 to 75 percent erection level and:

1. Grab your penis below the head and hold it out as if you were going to stretch. This will help stabilize your penis for the mini jelq.
2. Take your other hand and form a small pincher grip at the base of the smaller corpus chamber.
3. Using the small pincher grip, jelq the single chamber in a similar motion as you would a normal jelq. Your goal is to move the blood throughout that smaller corpus chamber. *Each mini jelq stroke should take two to three seconds.*

Straight Bends

Slinky bends and flaccid bends help fix a curve too (both described in Appendix C). Similar to the side jelq, perform the bends against the curve.

3. Becoming Multi-Orgasmic

Question: "Are there any penis exercises that can help me have multiple orgasms?"

Answer: Yes. You already know one of them: the kegel. When performed at the right time, the kegel can take you beyond overcoming premature ejaculation, beyond being able to last as long as you want, and into a new realm of sexual stamina: male multiple orgasms.[3]

Strong pelvic floor muscles—combined with lots of practice and the right timing—have turned quick shooters into no shooters. Dr. Barbara Keesling says in her easy-to-read book, *How to Make Love All Night*, "There are several steps to becoming multi-orgasmic, but building up the [pelvic floor muscles] is the crucial first step." Dr. Keesling adds, "Every man who is willing to do the work can bring his [pelvic floor muscles] to a state of readiness within two to three weeks. Often it takes even less than that."

How does the kegel help you have multiple orgasms? The trick, and the second step, is knowing and understanding your arousal. You have to become increasingly aware of your point of no return—the point where ejaculation is inevitable.

As you approach the point of no return, strong pelvic floor muscles are worth more than any thought about baseball stats, your grandmother naked, or any other image you pop into your head to delay an early discharge of the family seed. Here's why: It's common belief that ejaculation and orgasm are the same thing, but they are actually two different processes. They just typically come hand-in-hand. You can separate the two by doing a strong kegel—lasting roughly ten seconds or more—immediately before the point of no return. If done right, this will allow you to have an orgasm, but without ejaculating! As a result, your penis will still be aroused and erect.

The first few times you attempt using the kegel to stop ejaculation, you should do it by yourself, when you don't have the pressure of pleasing someone else. After you are able to have multiple orgasms on your own, try kegeling right before the point of no return when you are with a partner. Another thing you'll want to do, at least in the beginning, is stop all stimulation when you do the strong kegel. Meaning, if you are by yourself, stop stroking your penis. Then kegel. If you are with a partner, stop thrusting. Then kegel.

Also, for the first couple of times, it will probably be hard to hold back your ejaculation if you wait until right before the point of no return. So instead, build up to the point of no return. When you get to the point that you feel your arousal is fairly high—and that you'll ejaculate within a minute or two—stop and do a strong kegel. Let your arousal subside a bit and then restart. This time let your arousal build even higher, and then stop and kegel again.

Build up and stop five or six times, continually getting closer to the point of no return each time. Then, once you are at the point right before you orgasm, completely stop all stimulation, take a big deep breath, and kegel as hard as you possibly can. If everything goes according to plan, your body will go into orgasm without ejaculating, and you'll be able to go for Round 2.

Becoming multi-orgasmic often takes lots of practice. As one penis exerciser noted, "I started practicing to become multi-orgasmic about three months ago, and 100 ejaculations later I finally got it! . . . During the learning process, I experienced several sensations. On a few occasions, I even had an ejaculation, but no orgasm. It was weird, but it's really all part of learning how to separate the two."

A few pitfalls can hinder you from becoming multi-orgasmic. The main one is not having strong pelvic floor muscles. If this happens to you, spend a few weeks focusing extra-hard on your kegels (but don't over-train, or it will make it even more difficult). Another pitfall is not being completely in tune with your arousal or kegeling at the wrong time. If this occurs, make sure your body is completely relaxed. Take deep breaths and pay attention to all the sensations that you feel while building up to the point of no return.

4. Erection Difficulties

Question: "I'm still not harder. What's the problem?"

Answer: Numerous factors could be hindering your hardness. First, ask yourself the following questions. Are you focusing on the chief hardness exercises: the kegel, the jelq, and the stretch? Most importantly, are you really kegeling as much as you should? And if so, are you kegeling too much?

If you are sure that you are not over-training or under-training, then the strength of your erections might be spoiled by other causes, such as heart disease, an overall unhealthy lifestyle, and even stress.

Many men don't know that their emotions have a huge impact on their hardness. As Dr. Steven Lamm says in *The Hardness Factor*, "Depression, stress, and anxiety are significant inhibitors of libido (sex drive)." As more studies are conducted on hardness, it becomes evident that a happy outlook on life often provides a penis *full of life.*

"Not only does stress mar sexual performance, but the medications commonly used to treat it, such as anti-anxiety drugs, tend to depress the libido and inhibit desire," says Dr. Ian Kerner, sexologist and author of *She Comes First* and several other books. For instance, serotonin reuptake inhibitors (SSRIs)—such as Paxil, Prozac, and other anti-depressant drugs —increase the amount of serotonin in the brain. And extra serotonin has an adverse side effect of decreasing desire and libido, which results in decreasing hardness.

Bad health is also linked to weak erections. As Dr. Lamm points out, there is an "unmistakable link between failing erections and common medical ailments, including obesity, high cholesterol levels, hypertension, sleep disorders, diabetes, and heart disease."

Either stress or poor health could be the cause of your hardness troubles. Fortunately, you can do two things to fix both. First, if you believe the hardness problem to be largely associated with a serious problem (such as heart disease), seek medical attention immediately.

Second, strive to live an active, healthy, and happy lifestyle. Really focus on regularly exercising, eating well, and obtaining proper amounts of sleep. Also avoid cigarettes and large quantities of alcohol, as they too impede erection strength. Likewise, relax and enjoy the world you live in. These simple changes will make you and your penis healthy well into your retirement years; and combined with performing penis exercises, you should never have a problem maintaining a hard, solid erection.

5. Penis Supplements

Question: "Are there supplements to make the penis harder?"

Answer: Yes, several all-natural herbal supplements and vitamins can help produce a healthier, harder penis. "Using such nutritional powerhouses as Pycnogenol, L-arginine, omega-3 fatty acids, horny goat weed, and a host of antioxidant supplements, men can prevent and reverse most hardness problems," says Dr. Steven Lamm.

Along with promoting a healthier lifestyle, many of the following supplements will increase your erection strength and your libido.[4] As a side note, many of these supplements are also a great complement to performing penis exercises—not just for hardness, but also for enlargement. Contact your doctor before taking any of the following supplements. You can purchase these supplements and find out more information at most vitamin stores.

L-Arginine:

This amino acid enhances erection strength, pleasure, and sexual desire. L-arginine increases blood flow throughout the body and the penis, which is great for enlargement and even greater for hardness. Evidence suggests L-arginine's effects are dramatically enhanced when taken with Pycnogenol, another supplement that's effective at boosting hardness.

Omega-3 Fatty Acids:

These fatty acids play a key role in keeping the heart healthy. And the healthier your heart, the harder your erections. Evidence suggests that omega-3 fatty acids can substantially help reduce heart attacks and keep your heart fit and healthy, along with increasing sexual performance. The best food source for omega-3 is fish. Unfortunately, most of us don't get enough of omega-3 in our diets and need supplements to fulfill the void.

Horny Goat Weed:

This herbal supplement is infamous for increasing sexual desire and hardness. Its name comes from its antidote—it makes you horny.

Yohimbe:

For many men, yohimbe acts like nature's Viagra. It's a powerful stimulant, and therefore it shouldn't be taken daily. Instead, similar to Viagra, you take yohimbe an hour or two before a sexual encounter. (Note: Avoid this supplement if you have high blood pressure or any heart troubles).

Vitamins A, B, C and E:

All of these vitamins play a critical role in maintaining a healthy body, heart, and penis. The benefits of these vitamins are extensive, especially for hardness. They largely promote more blood flow to the penis as well as protect us against free radicals, which are connected to heart disease and weak erections. Most of these vitamins—along with other hardness boosting supplements—can be found in a single multivitamin.

6. Penis Enlargement Pills

Question: "Do penis enlargement pills work?"

Answer: You've probably seen the ads, or read the claims: *add two to four inches to your penis with a simple pill!* First, and foremost, I have found no evidence that validates any man enlarging his penis by taking a pill alone. My experience has been the opposite — I have talked to many men that have taken penis enlargement pills without gaining anything except more room in their wallet.

Nonetheless, the ingredients found in penis enlargement pills might be useful in *combination with penis exercises*. In fact, some penis exercisers have found them to be a great supplement to performing penis exercises. That said, many of the ingredients in penis enlargement pills can be found at a much cheaper price. If you're looking for an extra boost in your gains, look into taking supplements such as whey protein, L-arginine, horny goat weed, and a daily multivitamin.

7. Gaining Troubles

Question: "I've tried everything and I still can't gain. What's the problem?"

Answer: When it comes to penis enlargement growth, there are four kinds of gainers. The first gainer is the guy who gains both length and girth easily. He obtains his goal the quickest. The next two gainers are either length gainers or girth gainers. These men gain easily in a specific area (such as girth) and lack gains in the other area (such as length). These guys typically reach their easy goal first, and then specifically target the other area. The last gainer is the hard gainer. He has to work extra hard to reach his goal.

Before you condemn yourself as a hard gainer, realize that enlarging the penis—like the muscles—takes time. Your biceps won't double in size (no matter how much you exercise) in just a few months, and your penis won't either.

That said, some guys hit the gym day after day only to get the same unchanging results. They don't lose weight, they don't gain muscle, and the only shape they get in is round. Unfortunately, some men also perform penis exercises day after day with similar unsatisfying results. The reason for these poor results are often caused by many of the principles covered in this book, such as not obtaining enough rest, not increasing the intensity, or increasing the intensity too much.

Poor results, however, might just be caused by simple genetics.

Just as some men can't gain weight or muscle mass if their life depended on it, other men have the toughest time enlarging their penis—largely for reasons out of their control. Nonetheless, regardless of what is inhibiting your gains, in my experience there's always one thing that produces penis enlargement growth: persistence.

If you tried everything in this book, then my final recommendation is first stop doing whatever you've been doing. It's not working. Take a two to four month break. It might be hard to convince yourself that taking a break helps, but your penis needs to return to its pre-penis exercises state. Once you return, start out light and completely change it up. Try new things. Change the amount of days you exercise, the amount of force you use, and the kind of exercises you do. Exercise for less amount of time and with less force first, then try more time and more force. Do everything and anything.

Go the next step and change your lifestyle, which has worked for some hard gainers. For example, if you're a smoker, then quit. If you don't regularly exercise at the gym, then start. Eat healthy too. Even more important, try some of the supplements and vitamins suggested in the previous question. If all else fails, you might consider using a penis enlargement device. You could also go to one of the websites in Appendix D, where you will find more specific advice on what other men did to jump start their gains.

8. Penis Enlargement Devices

Question: "What is a penis enlargement device? What are the common devices? Are they expensive? Are they safe?"

Answer: A penis enlargement device is an appliance that does the penis exercises for you. Penis enlargement devices often yield effective results, especially when combined with traditional penis exercises. The common devices include penile hangers, penile pumps, all day stretchers, extenders, clamping devices, and jelq simulators. Some devices—such as hangers and all day stretchers—can be used throughout the day with minimal effort.

Devices are also useful if you're having a hard time gaining, or if you want to kick-start growth. Many men start using a device after they are comfortable performing penis exercises or once they hit a plateau.

> **NOTE:** Because this book's focus is on penis exercises and not penis enlargement devices, this section is just an overview of the most common devices. Do not use a device without consulting the manufacturer or another resource. Most importantly, do not use this section as your sole information on devices. There's enough information to be said about devices to serve another book. If after performing penis exercises for several months you want to try using a device, then go to http://www.PEGym.com/devices. There you will find more information on how to use each device, pictures of the devices in use, and a directory of the current penis enlargement devices.

"What Are the Common Devices?"

Penis Hanger:

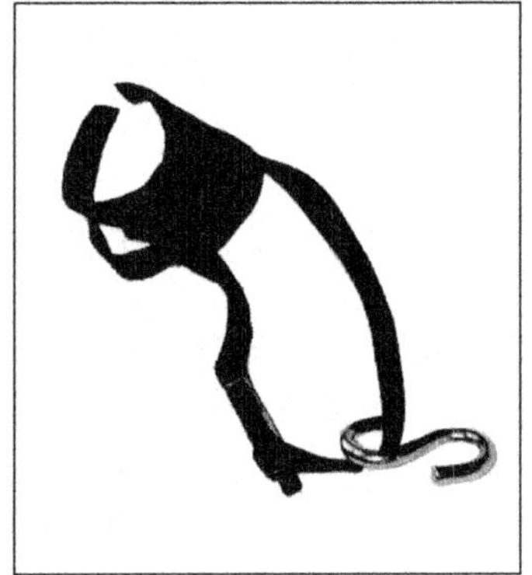

Penis Hanger

This device is an advanced type of stretching and is most useful for acquiring length. One end of the device attaches to some part of your penis shaft (not the head) and the other end hangs weight. Many penis enlargement surgeons recommend using a hanger after surgery. With hanging, the amount of weight and time used varies greatly. Weight can range from less than a pound to thirty pounds or more. Hanging high weight from the penis is often unnecessary and isn't advised for beginners. Time can range from less than an hour to several hours or more.

All Day Stretcher:

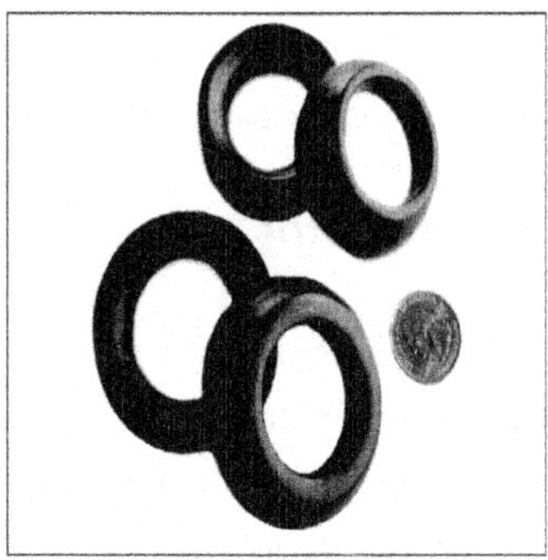
All Day Stretcher

This is a light hanger-type device that is used for long periods of time. An all day stretcher (ADS) has the benefit of keeping the penis in a stretched state and is typically used in combination with a hanger. Some men, for example, use a typical hanger for a few hours and then use an ADS for the rest of the day. A popular all day stretching method involves hanging extremely light weights, known as Penis Exercise Weights (shown to the right), on the penis. The penis slides through the weights, and a piece of cloth is used to keep the weights in place. Like most effective all day stretchers, Penis Exercise Weights are fairly stealthy and can be worn in public.

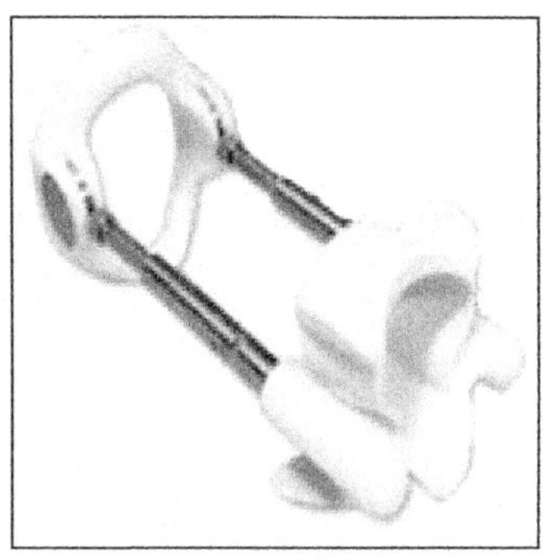
Extender

Extender:

This is a unique device in that it can generally be used by beginners right away and requires very little work. It is a stretching device that keeps the penis extended throughout the day, and is hidden underneath your clothes so no one can tell that you are wearing it. Extenders are one of the few penis exercises methods that have gone under several clinical trials, and thus are one of the most popular devices. They work by having one side encircle the base of the penis and the other side stretch out the penis. Along with being a useful supplement to standard penis exercises, extenders are also

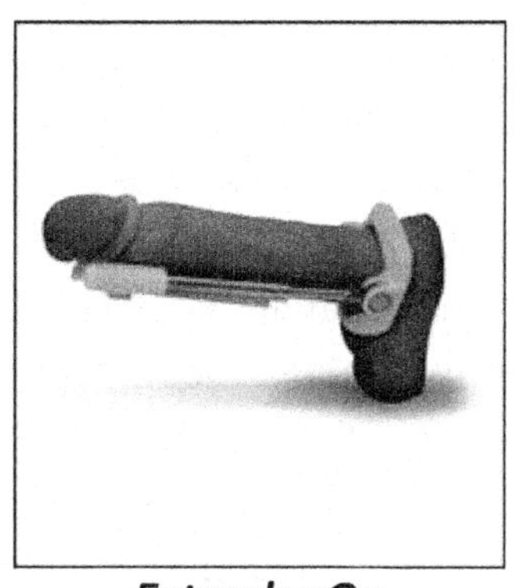
Extender On

useful for increasing flaccid size. Some doctors declare that extenders can also fix Peyronie's disease—a severe and often painful curve.[6]

Jelq Simulator

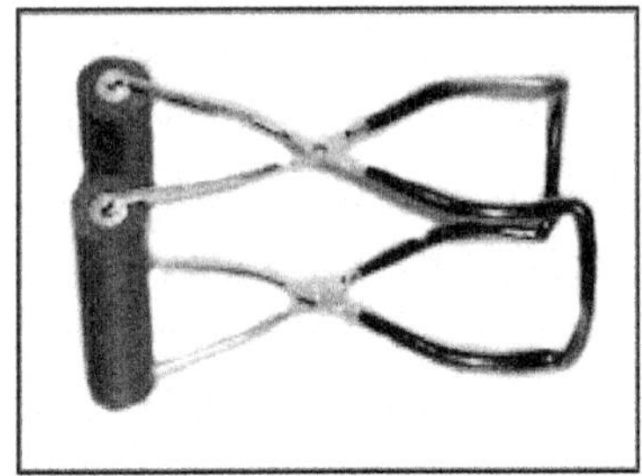

Jelq Simulator

This device is designed to provide the same effect as the jelq, but with more intensity and consistency. Most jelq simulators, like the Jelq Device shown to the right, use two padded cylinders to jelq the penis. Jelq simulators are practical in that they increase the intensity of the jelq while giving your hands a break. They also don't require the use of a lubricant, so they make clean up easy and hassle free.

Penis Pump:

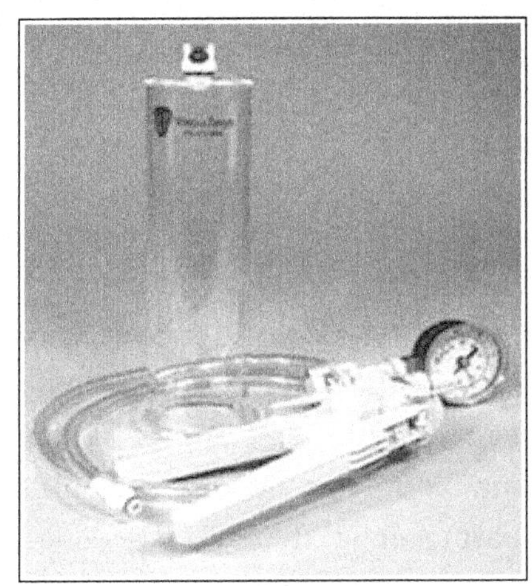

Penis Pump

This is the most popular penis enlargement device. Penile pumps have been used to make the penis harder and temporarily bigger for decades. Using a penile pump, or pumping, involves placing the penis in a vacuum cylinder tube. Once inside the tube, pressure is added to *pump the penis up.* For sex, you place your penis in the tube until it is hard enough for penetration. For penis enlargement, you place the penis in the pump for several minutes or more. Although the results from pumping are often temporary, many men have acquired permanent gains when using a penile pump combined with the traditional penis exercises.

Originally, the penis was pumped using a hand pump. Recently, electrical pumps—which do all the work for you—have hit the market. Both electrical and hand pumps are effective. Penile pumps are sold at most adult novelty stores, online stores, and sex catalogs. The best pumps have a pressure gauge. Without a pressure gauge, you can easily go overboard.

Clamping Device:

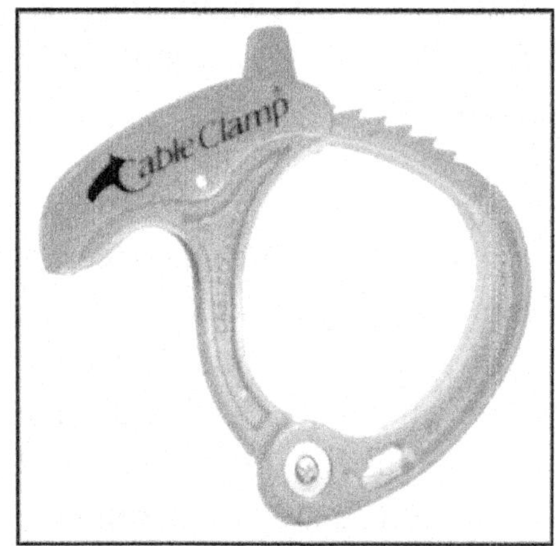

Modified Clamping Device

This device works by clamping off the base of the penis for a short period of time. Clamping devices inhibit blood from leaving the penis, which increases penile blood pressure and causes the penis to expand the only way it can: outward. Clamping is similar to the uli exercise (described in Appendix C), but entails using a tight cock ring or any other kind of constricting device. The picture on the right is of a Cable Clamp, which many men use in conjunction with soft padding. Although clamping is fairly new, it has allowed many men to significantly expand their girth. That said, many men have found that it's easy to go overboard with clamping, and several of the self-prescribed penile Mondor's disease cases are often due to clamping.

"Are Devices Expensive?"

Devices vary in price—ranging from just a few dollars to well into the hundreds. The least expensive route is to build a device yourself. Instructions for building penis enlargement devices can be found at several of the websites in Appendix D, many of which also have information on purchasing devices.

The more expensive route is to purchase a device, which requires more money, but less work. The most expensive devices include the majority of hangers, extenders, and pumps. Most hangers cost roughly 100 dollars or more. Penile pumps cost around 100 dollars for a hand pump and typically well over 500 dollars for an electrical pump. Extenders generally cost 150 dollars or more.

Jelq simulators, all day stretchers, and clamps are all on the lower end of the price spectrum. Most jelq simulators cost less than 100 dollars. Some all day stretchers, such as Penis Exercise weights, cost less than fifteen dollars. Most clamping devices are sold at a retail stores for less than five dollars.

"Are Devices Safe?"

Safety is often a concern—and rightfully so—when using a device. Penis enlargement devices can be both scary and dangerous. They are, however, generally safe if you use a secure device, common sense, and the proper guidelines. The real danger lies within not knowing your limits. You can easily go overboard and add more weight than you need with a hanger, or use more pressure than you need with a pump. (Common sense tells you that you shouldn't start out hanging more than a pound or two from your penis.) The darkening effect is also more likely to occur when using a device—especially clamping.

If safety is a major concern, consider the fact that several doctors instruct the use of a penile hanger or pump after penis enlargement surgery. Nevertheless, if you decide to use a device, it's even more essential that you follow all the guidelines outlined throughout this book. Also follow these device-safety principles:

Follow a strict time limit:

In the beginning, use clamping devices, pumps, and hangers for a maximum of ten minutes at a time. Overtime, you can move up to a maximum of twenty minutes, but no longer. Your penis needs to obtain proper amounts of blood flow to stay hard and healthy, and most devices limit circulation. After each set, give your penis at least ten minutes to recuperate. All day stretchers and extenders can be worn for longer periods of time without rest, but still take them off for a few moments every so often.

Use wrapping for protection, comfort, and support when able:

Many hangers, all day stretchers, and clamping devices are built so you can wrap your penis with a soft fabric underneath the device. You can use any cloth-like material to wrap, including a sock, a strip of mouse pad, Homedics magnetic wrap, or Ace's bandage—most of which can be found at any retail store, such as Walmart. Using a wrap will not only protect your penis, it will also help keep the skin of your penis looking nice and healthy.

Never let a hanger, stretcher, or any other device hang from the head of your penis: The head is the most sensitive part of your penis and thus the most prone to injury.

Constantly monitor your penis temperature and color:

If your penis feels cold or turns dark blue, purple, or black, immediately remove the device. In either instance, your penis is starving for fresh oxygenated blood, which is essential for your penis' health. After the device is removed, do ten kegels and jelqs to push fresh blood into your penis.

Always start out extremely light and work your way up:

This principle applies tenfold when using a device, because you don't have as much control as you do when using your hands. With your hands, you can stop at any moment. With a device, however, it could take anywhere from seconds to minutes to remove the device. These few seconds can seem like a lifetime in the instance that something goes wrong. Moreover, it's really easy to push your penis way beyond its limits with a device—especially with hanging and clamping, which are the two devices most prone to cause an injury. The safest way to use a penis enlargement device is to start out well below what you think you can handle. Start with low weight, pressure, and time.

If you diligently follow these guidelines, you will dramatically minimize the chances of anything wrong occurring. For more safety principles on each particular device, go to the device manufacturer.

9. Penis Enlargement Surgery

Question: "Is there penis enlargement surgery?"

Answer: Yes. Many men who don't know of penis exercises, or who don't have the time or patience to commit to a program, decide to go under the knife.

Unfortunately, penis enlargement surgery isn't as successful as breast enlargement surgery, and the results are often disappointing. In a recent study published by St. Peter's Andrology Centre and Institute of Urology, urologist David Ralph and colleagues reported that most men who underwent penis enlargement surgery weren't pleased with the results. In fact, out of forty-two men, only "thirty-five percent of the men were satisfied with the outcome."

The surgery involved cutting out the penile ligaments, which is the most common technique. Other techniques include silicon injection, using inflatable implants, and grafting fat from other parts of the body into the penis.

"The operation does lengthen the flaccid penis, but usually only by one centimeter (which is just under a half an inch)," says Ralph and his colleagues in the European Urology. Yet, "some patients who persevere with post-op stretching exercises, as much as three centimeters can be achieved, but patients must also be warned that a small degree of penile shortening may occur."

On the other hand, Dr. Douglas Whitehead, president of the American Academy of Phalloplasty Surgeons and a leading penis enlargement surgeon, suggests a better outcome is more likely. "The average expected length gain is one inch. But well motivated patients may gain up to two inches," says Whitehead. Dr. Gary Alter, another leading doctor in penis enlargement surgery, says, "Length increases of several inches are rare . . . however, some compulsive weight-hanging users report gains of several inches."

Whatever the case, it's clear the men who use a penis enlargement hanger after surgery gain much more than the men who don't. It's also clear that penis enlargement surgery has had mixed reviews. For this reason, several urologists still condemn penis enlargement surgery, and only suggest it when it's absolutely necessary (and it usually isn't). Moreover, the results of surgery are often temporary—especially the results of the girth procedures.

The moderators of the Yahoo! Group: Surgical Enlargement Forum, which oversee 5000 members interested in penis enlargement surgery, declare, "Girth enhancement as it is practiced today has not proven successful in spite of what those offering it tell you."

Dr. Patrick Hudson is an example of many surgeons who don't perform penis enlargement surgery. "There are several risks that might take place, including infection, scarring, numbness, and loss of penile function."

Nevertheless, anyone who is thinking about undertaking penis enlargement surgery should do thorough research beforehand. As they say, "you get what you pay for;" and when shopping for the right surgeon, the cheap route is most likely not the safe route. Some doctors are better than others, and there have been a few horror stories of men who had nothing but complications after penis enlargement surgery, often because they didn't go with an experienced doctor. If you are considering surgery as an option, do your research, contact past patients of each doctor, and don't do it until you know what to expect.

Dr. Hudson advises, "There are no state or federal laws that control how doctors are trained in penis enlargement surgery, and anyone can call themselves an expert! You may want to look for a board certified surgeon who specializes in penis enlargement surgery."

At any rate, the effectiveness and safety of penis enlargement surgery is actually getting better. In anywhere from ten to twenty years, penis enlargement surgery might become so successful that it will be as common as breast enlargement surgery.

10. Increasing Flaccid Size

Question: "How can I increase the size of my flaccid penis?"

Answer: If one of your main reasons for penis exercises is to enlarge your flaccid penis, you're not alone. Many men care about the size of their flaccid penis more than they do their erect size. Perhaps your reasoning is simply for prowess and showing—when you're in the locker room, at a nude beach, or when you're wearing your disco pants from the 70s. Or perhaps you're trying to create the "full package" for your partner, and a penis that is larger and fuller-looking is sometimes more gratifying to both men and women. One woman I interviewed told me, "I don't care about the size of a penis when it's erect. It's the sight of a large bulge in a man's pants that really turns me on."

Regardless of your reasoning, your flaccid size will generally increase as your erect penis size does. It might even grow before your erect size does, which is a health body clue and a sign of future erect growth. Some men find, however, that no matter how much their erect size grows, they are unable to increase their flaccid size with traditional exercises.

For instance, one man added over three inches to his erect size, which put him above eight inches in erect length. Yet he was still sporting the same flaccid size before he started performing penis exercises: less than three inches. Fortunately, there are several things that can be done to increase flaccid size. By improving the quality of his blood flow and keeping his penis in an extended state throughout the day, the man reports that he is now a "shower," with his flaccid penis nearly the same size has his erect. You can do the same too.

Improving Blood Flow

If you want to increase your flaccid size, focus on improving blood flow to your nether regions. Not only will this help you optimize the size of your flaccid hang, it will also optimize your penis health. To improve your blood flow, follow all the advice in Chapter 13: Look Bigger, Feel

Bigger. Also:

- Do your kegels frequently. Get a solid workout in at least three to four times a week.
- Drink plenty of water. Shoot for at least half of your body weight in ounces. So if you weigh 180 pounds, drink 90 or more ounces of water daily.
- Take the supplements recommended in the Penis Supplements section of Appendix A. Many men have reported good results with L-arginine, omega-3 fatty acids, and ginseng.
- Rub Essential Vein Oil or another mixture with vasodilators on your penis once or twice a day.
- Try going commando. Several men have reported that throwing caution to the wind and letting their family jewels live freely have helped improve circulation.
- Above all, avoid things that decrease blood flow: caffeine, drugs, cigarettes, and large quantities of alcohol (although a daily glass of wine might actually help *improve* blood flow).

Avoiding caffeine is important, as it curls up the little guy as quickly as a swift kick to the groin. Caffeine is a vasoconstrictor, which decreases blood flow throughout your body and penis. Countless men have noticed a dramatic increase in their flaccid size just by skipping the morning caffeine boost.

"I always heard that caffeine was bad for my penis health and size, but I never believed it until recently," said one man. "I went on a family vacation for two weeks. I was limited to one cup of coffee a day, opposed to my normal four to six. I noticed an immediate effect on my flaccid size and so did the wife. Not only did she notice my bulge, she thought I was erect. That ended up being a great night!" If you need a daily boost without caffeine, try other natural supplements like vitamin B and ginseng.

Never Let Your Penis Turtle

Along with keeping good blood flow, you'll want to follow the advice of a man who uses the online alias Big Girtha: "never let it turtle." He was referring to the *turtling* effect, when the penis deflates to a 0 percent erection level. By avoiding it like the plague he has increased his flaccid size by several inches and helped countless men follow in his footsteps.

How can you avoid the turtling effect? By keeping your flaccid penis in an extended or engorged state for a long period of time. You can do this several ways.

To keep the penis engorged throughout the day, try wearing a penis ring or a magnetic wrist wrap. Tightly secure the wrap or the ring at the base of your penis. This minimizes blood from leaving your penis, causes it to fill with more blood, and thus causes your penis to expand. Penis rings can be found at most adult shops, and magnetic wrist wraps can be found at most large pharmacies.

With penis rings, wrist wraps, and anything else you use to keep the penis engorged, keep in mind that the idea is to have maximum blood flow in the penis. After you get the device on, do a few Kegels and stimulate your penis here and there to keep the circulation going. Also, be sure that there is still some blood flowing into and out of the penis, as your penis needs fresh oxygen to survive. If it turns dark or feels numb, you have it on too tight.

To keep your penis in an extended statc, try wearing an all day stretcher or a penis extender (see the Penis Enlargement Devices section for more information on these devices). You can also try doing fowfers.

Fowfer

A natural exercise that keeps your penis extended and doesn't require purchasing a device is the "fowfer," which is named after the online alias of the man who created them. He reports that it helped him go from a "grower" to a "shower" in a few months, and many men have reported similar results by doing this simple exercise on a daily basis.

The fowfer requires no hands and is done while you're sitting down. As long as you can find a second of privacy to get situated, you'll be free to do other things and the world will never know the difference. To do the fowfer, make sure your erection level is in the 10 to 40 percent range. Then:

3. Place the head of your penis on the outside of your anus or near it. The hole provides an extra cushion so there shouldn't be any pressure on your head. You can also place your penis under one of your cheeks.
4. Carefully sit down. Your penis should be in a fixed, stretched position. There shouldn't be any pain or discomfort.
5. Stay in the fowfer position for anywhere from 10 to 120 minutes. Many men find that 10 to 20 minutes is enough, some men need longer. Either way, release the fowfer every 20 minutes and massage your penis to get the blood flowing again.

Whether you use a fowfer, a device, or even just manual exercises, you'll want to avoid doing too much, as it generally causes your flaccid penis to turtle for long periods of time.

11. Premature Ejaculation

Question: "Is there anything I can do to combat premature ejaculation?"

Answer: Let's face it, next to a small penis, premature ejaculation has to rank at the top of worries for a lot of men. Even the most sensitive partner can grow frustrated with a "minute man." Technically, premature ejaculation is defined as uncontrolled ejaculation before or shortly after sexual penetration, before the man wishes, and often with minimal sexual stimulation. It is one of the most common forms of sexual dysfunction in guys, and has affected almost every man at least once in his life. Using penis exercises can help you control premature ejaculation in three steps:

- Step 1 – Create pelvic floor balance, through the use of kegels;
- Step 2 – Understand the concept of arousal; and
- Step 3 – Practice makes perfect.

Step 1 – Create Pelvic Floor Balance through the use of Kegels

Although the cause of premature ejaculation is often unclear, creating pelvic floor balance is key to have rock hard and long-lasting erections. When there is too much high tone (tension) or too much low tone (weakness) in the pelvic floor muscles, an imbalance occurs. If you have too much tension, this can lead to involuntary kegels leading to premature ejaculation. If you have weakness in the pelvic floor muscles, this can lead to a complete lack of involuntary kegels, which leads to delayed ejaculation. Instead, what you want is balance in these muscles, without too much tension and without weakness, so you can control when you ejaculate.

Involuntary kegels aren't necessarily a bad thing. They are critical in reaching orgasm and facilitate ejaculation. However, the goal is to develop your muscles so involuntary kegels don't happen before you want them to. Instead, you want to be able to suppress this involuntary urge, until you're ready to orgasm.

How to Identify an Unbalanced Pelvic Floor:

There are several ways to help identify an unbalanced pelvic floor. These include:

- Premature ejaculation,
- Delayed ejaculation,
- Poor erection quality,
- Reduced libido,
- Uncontrollable kegels/spasms,
- Incontinence,
- Difficulty urinating and defecating,
- Pain in the pelvic floor region, or
- Hardness when flaccid.

How to Bring Your Pelvic Floor Muscles Into Balance:

For those with too much tension in their pelvic floor muscles – reverse kegels, pelvic stretches, relaxation techniques, and massage are key. Your penis exercise routine should consist of 60 to 70 percent reverse kegels, with the remainder being regular kegels. In fact, you may want to begin with only doing reverse kegels for the first couple of weeks.

If you experience pelvic floor weakness, then you'll want to have a kegel routine based on at least 50 percent of your routine including regular kegels. Whether you have too much tension or weakness, the end goal is the same – healthy, strong and balanced pelvic floor muscles. Where kegels are a conscious contraction of the BC and IC muscles, reverse kegels (as the name implies) is the opposite. Reverse kegels are a purposeful relaxing of these muscles.

Step 2 – Understand the Concept of Arousal

Arousal occurs when the brain releases chemicals known as *endorphins.* Endorphins are natural painkillers that have a similar chemical structure to that of heroin and other opiates. According to Dr. Barbra Keesling, if you build your sexual arousal in a predictable way, you can release a large amount of endorphins, over a period of time. To develop arousal awareness, Dr. Keesling suggests using an arousal scale, consisting of three levels.

- **Level 1: "Gentle"** - This occurs at the early stage of arousal. You know you're aroused, but don't feel you have to do anything about it. You can just enjoy the feeling of being aroused. The lower end of this level includes not being aroused at all.
- **Level 2: Strong** – This, according to Dr. Keesling is a more active, insistent arousal. You feel like you want to act on the feeling, either with a partner or alone.
- **Level 3: Urgent** – Level 3 arousal includes a driving need that you respond to the feeling. Your arousal demands your attention, and it can take you over the edge into orgasm at the highest end of this level.[7]

The key here is to listen to your body. Although it may be tempting to lose yourself in the moment, always be aware of your arousal level, whether with a partner or performing penis exercises. As you begin to climb toward Level 3, pay attention to these feelings, and bring yourself back down to a safe Level 2.

Step 3 – Practice Makes Perfect

The old saying "Practice makes perfect." is very true when it comes to performing penis exercises to help prevent premature ejaculation. Consistency is key. Practice, practice, practice! Whether you're using kegels or the other exercises listed below, try to work up to 20-minute sessions. Increasing your stamina while exercising will help you increase your stamina in the bedroom.

Additionally, don't ejaculate every time you exercise. Again, listen to your body and learn the cues your body gives before you orgasm. When you start to feel yourself reaching this point of no return, back off.

Lastly, start your exercising sessions with positive affirmations. Tell yourself you can do this and believe it. Having the right mental frame of mind is crucial! If you go into the exercises thinking you can't last, you're setting yourself up for failure. A positive attitude and believing in yourself will get you on the path to success.

Kegels for Premature Ejaculation Treatment

As noted earlier in this chapter, kegels have numerous benefits. From building a harder and larger penis and improving prostate health, to increasing ejaculation volume and producing stronger orgasms, kegels are critical to male sexual health. In the case of premature ejaculation, kegels strengthen your PC muscle, and once your PC muscle is strong, it can help you control the urge to ejaculate.

For kegels to work for premature ejaculation, you must be able to hold the contraction for at least ten seconds. When you're able to do this, try the following to help delay orgasm:

- Kegel right before you reach the point of no return,
- Hold the contraction for at least ten seconds, and
- Once the urge to ejaculate has passed, release the kegel.

Training your PC muscle to be strong enough to withstand the pressure of ejaculation is the hardest part of this solution. Training can take anywhere from several weeks to years. Once you've strengthened your PC muscle, you'll also need to know when to do the kegel. Timing, as they say, is everything.

PEGym.com Member Premature Ejaculation Success Stories

Member Name: ethan1066

ethan1066 described premature ejaculation as both disgusting and frustrating. To get over this challenge, he had great success with cock rings. He noted that the pressure slowed the flow of blood leaving from the erect penis, which resulted in not only a harder erection, but significantly increased his stamina.

Member Name: Omegablue

Omegablue had been edging for awhile, but had just started jelqing and ballooning. After only a week, he noticed a significant difference in how much his stamina had increased. The exercises, plus relaxation techniques helped him increase how long he lasted with his girlfriend, from three minutes to over 20 minutes! Omegablue said, "I tried relaxing the whole entire time and when I got to the PONR, I would just totally relax and breathe."

He noted that the head of his cock always felt over sensitive, when he had sex. To counter this, while ballooning, he rubbed the head on and off to help desensitize it. This, along with the relaxation, has helped him control when he orgasms.

Member Name: RyboT

RyboT took the matter of premature ejaculation into his own hands – literally. He used masturbation to help overcome premature ejaculation. He noted, "Instead of going for the gold straight away, I now see how long I can go for without feeling the urge to cum." Thanks to this hands-on experience building, RyboT has extended his time by at least ten minutes and says he can now cum pretty much on demand.

Member Name: Carson32

Carson32 found the opposite solution to be true, when compared to RyboT. His masturbation habit had conditioned himself to cum as quickly as possible. He stopped masturbating so frequently and re-trained his ejaculatory reflex to last longer than his original 30 seconds.

Member Name: HighHopes

HighHopes found that he had a problem with premature ejaculation, especially when a day or two had passed without having sex with his girlfriend. He would feel like ejaculating after only one or two penetrations. His solution was reverse kegels. When he felt too excited during sex, he'd relax, perform reverse kegels and keep going. HighHopes was able to use reverse kegels to pace himself so that he could finally cum at the same time as his girlfriend, which was not only a huge relief but also a tremendous confidence booster.

Member Name: trainingtzr

After hearing how is girlfriend's ex lasted significantly longer than he did in bed, traningtzr knew he had to do something about his premature ejaculation. He found several things helped. First, he tried to keep his mind off of sex before the actual event and concentrated on foreplay for his girlfriend. Once having sex, he used distraction, by thinking of random, non-stimulating topics, to keep his arousal level down. When he began to reach the PONR, trainingtzr also found reverse kegels to help control his arousement level.

Member Name: Panther

Panther suffered from premature ejaculation for many years. He attributed it to a "screwed up childhood." He found five steps to solving his problem:

1. Kegels, kegels, kegels;
2. Breathing from the lower belly and relaxation;
3. He reduced his anxiety by talking with his girlfriend, telling her the problem and having her commit to helping him;
4. He learned to enjoy the journey of sex as much as the orgasmic ending; and

5. He sought counseling for the issues he needed to address in his childhood.

Member Name: michaela

michaela suffered from premature ejaculation, and still occasionally does. He found that premature ejaculation for him centered on learned behavior from masturbation and previous sexual experiences, which led to quick release. These resulted in a conditioned behavior that sex meant cum quickly. He changed his masturbation techniques and also realized he needed to work on his anxiety levels.

The anxiety levels were his biggest roadblock. When he was anxious, he found his body was automatically in tense mode. His muscles were contracted and his breathing was heavy. Both of these are counter-productive to increasing your stamina.

Appendix B:

The Penis Anatomy

Throughout this book, the anatomy jargon is kept to a minimum so that everyone—regardless of their anatomy knowledge—can build a solid foundation of how to perform penis exercises. But many men find that once they start performing penis exercises, they want to know more about how their favorite organ really works. So, here it is: the penis uncovered and exposed, as you've never seen it before.[9]

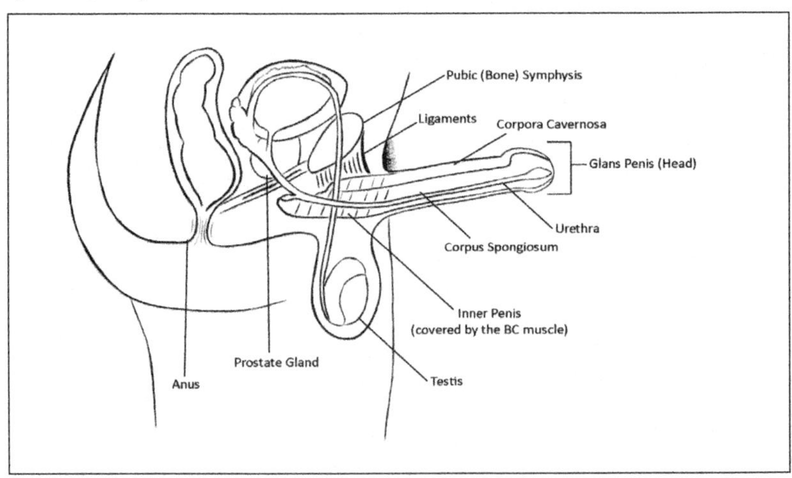

Figure 1: Side View of the Penis

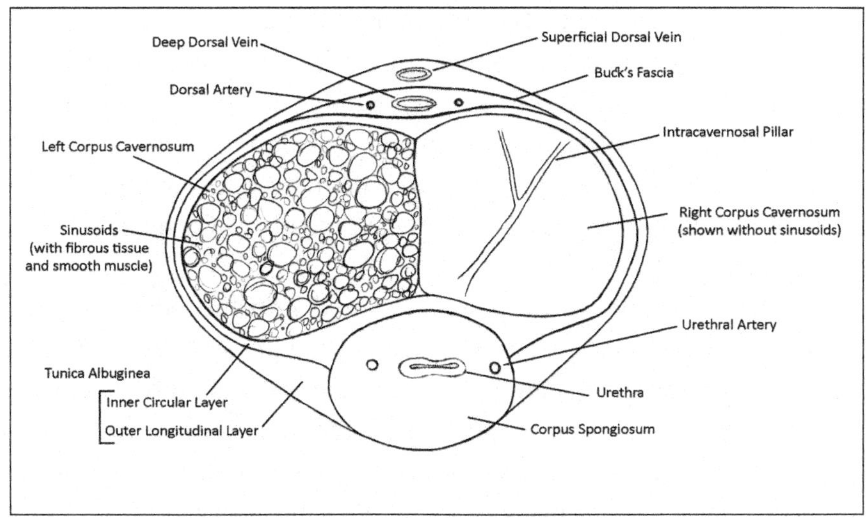

Figure 2: Three Corpus Chambers

The Penis

The penis is like the rest of our body. For the most part, we have a basic sense of what everything is, but don't exactly know how and why it all works. The penis is a complex organ composed of many different tissues, including ligaments, skeletal muscle, smooth muscle, veins, arteries, and other tissues that cooperate in perfect harmony when your penis goes from flaccid to erect, and vice versa.

The Three Corpus Chambers

The main body of the penis is composed of three circular chambers. Together, the top two chambers make up the corpora cavernosa. The bottom chamber holds the urethra and makes up the corpus spongiosum. All three chambers are largely composed of smooth muscle and collagen—a protein that forms the connective tissue within the penis. The mini jelq—an exercise designed to fix a penis curve—focuses on jelqing only one of the top corpus cavernosum chambers.

The Pelvic Floor Muscles

Most men think of the penis as a completely external organ. But when you stand naked in the mirror, you're only seeing half of the picture. The other half of your penis extends inside your body—and is known as the inner penis. Your inner penis is encircled by and composed of the pelvic floor muscles—largely the bulbocavernosus (BC) muscle and the ischiocavernosus (IC) muscle.

Together, the two muscles pump blood into the penis, causing a chain reaction that leads to an erection. These muscles are vital to a healthy genital region. Fortunately, kegeling keeps these muscles in shape.

You can feel the inner penis and the pelvic floor muscles by touching your perineum—the area between your testicles and your anus. Sex pioneer Dr. Alfred Kinsey noticed that the perineum is "highly sensitive to touch, and tactile stimulation of the area may provide considerable erotic arousal." This sensitivity is most likely due to the fact that you are actually rubbing your penis (the inner portion of it). You are also rubbing your prostate, which is on the other side of your pelvic floor muscles.

Arteries and Veins

Whereas the pelvic floor muscles pump blood into the penis, the arteries and veins provide the plumbing for the blood to get in and out. The penis has many penile arteries and veins. The most prominent being the dorsal vein and dorsal artery, located on the top part of the penis. The majority of the veins are on the outside of the corpus chambers. The majority of the arteries take a direct route inside the chambers.

The placement of the veins and arteries are a critical part of the erection process. When you become aroused, the arteries inside the chambers pump the penis full of blood. Once the penis is full of blood, the veins are pressed against the tunica, which stops blood from leaving the penis so you can maintain a hard, strong erection. If your pelvic floor muscles are weak, or if you have heart trouble or any other medical ailment that causes poor blood flow, your penis won't fill up with enough blood to press the veins against the tunica. This leads to a viscous cycle of blood quickly going into the penis, but leaving just as quickly—which causes erectile dysfunction.

The Smooth Muscle

Located inside the three corpus chambers, the smooth muscle cells help form the shape and size of your penis. When the smooth muscle is contracted, the penis is in its flaccid state. When the smooth muscle relaxes, the corpus chambers fill with blood, and an erection takes place. Healthy smooth muscle is essential to the overall well-being of the penis and its erections. "Complete smooth muscle relaxation is both necessary and sufficient to [obtain] an erection," says Dr. George J. Christ in an article published in Urologic Clinics of North America. And studies suggest that men who have low amounts of smooth muscle (generally less than 40 percent) have higher incidents of erectile dysfunction.

The Tunica

Once the smooth muscle relaxes, it presses against the tunica. The tunica is a strong tendon-like tissue that surrounds all three corpus chambers—and the smooth muscle within the chambers. Medically known as tunica albuginea, the tunica is actually an extension of the pelvic floor muscles. Peyronie's disease—a painful curve—is caused by plaque and fibrosis in the tunica.

The tunica typically consists of two layers: the inner circular layer and the outer longitudinal layer. The inner circular layer serves to govern the size of the erect penis similar to how a bicycle tire limits the expansion of the inner tube inside. As with a bike tire, once the limit of the tunica is reached, further pressure results in stiffness rather than expansion. Along with the intracavernosal pillars, the inner circular layer of the tunica holds up the corpus chambers. The outer longitudinal layer encircles all the corpus chambers together and functions to regulate the length of the expanding penis.

Oddly enough, not every man has the same amount of layers of tunica. Some men only have one layer in their penis. Others have as much as three layers. Some people speculate that the men who have a hard time gaining might have three layers of tunica, whereas the easy gainers might only have one layer. For the penis to enlarge, the tunica presumably needs to enlarge too; and a thicker tunica is in all likelihood harder to stretch than a thinner one.

The Glans

The head of the penis is also known as the glans. Housing an abundance of nerves, the head is the most sensitive part of your body. Inside the glans is a tough ligament known as the distal ligament. This hard ligament is a continuation of the tunica and acts as a coating for the glans, which makes the tip of the penis hard enough to penetrate the vagina during sex.

When born, the male glans is covered with a coat of skin that is cut off (circumcised) in many Western countries. The benefits and risks of circumcision have been under harsh debate in recent years, with the medical community at war on whether the procedure causes permanent harm physically and mentally for a child. Some believe that circumcision decreases sensitivity in the penis, and a few men have gone as far as

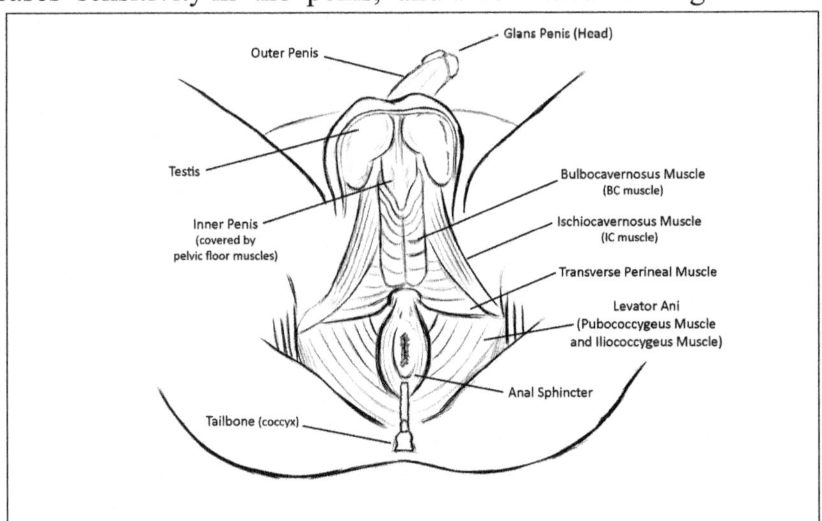

Figure 3: Pelvic Floor Muscles

hanging a particularly type of weight device from their penis in an effort to grow back their foreskin. Others believe that the whole debate is nonsense. Clive Peters, author of *How to Maximize Your Manhood: What every red-blooded male needs to know*, says, "Contrary to what you might think, there is little or no difference in sensitivity between cut and uncut men.*"*

The Ligaments

To keep your penis and scrotum properly stabilized, there are two main ligaments that attach to the penis: the fundiform ligament and the suspensory ligament. Both ligaments are located near the pubic bone. The suspensory ligament attaches the pubic bone to the penis in a web-like manner. The fundiform ligament comes from the lower abdomen, and encircles both the penis and scrotum.

The ligaments are cut during penis enlargement surgery, which exposes more of the inner penis—the part of the penis that is inside the body. Stretching downward similarly stretches the ligaments, also turning more of the inner penis into outer penis.

The Mechanism Behind Penis Enlargement and the Factors that Limit Enlargement

We've talked, in depth, about the anatomy of the penis, but it's important to understand the mechanics behind why penis enlargement works as well as the physical factors of your penis that limit enlargement, to get the most of your penis enlargement efforts. As we noted earlier, your penis consists of three chambers:

- Two chambers of the *corpus spongiosum* and
- One chamber of the *corpus cavernosum.*

When blood flows into the chambers, your penis becomes erect.

The chambers are separated by a thick band of connective tissue, called the *tunica albuginea.* This gives your penis the elasticity it needs to expand, when it's erect, and contract when it's flaccid. It's this elasticity, and being able to stretch the *tunica albuginea* more so the penis can grow larger, that is so important in penis enlargement.

The challenge is that the *tunica albuginea* is made up of not only elastic tissue, but also collagen. Collagen is an extremely tough connective tissue, used in the body to give structural strength to parts. Body parts like tendons and ligaments are made of collagen, as is most of our body's structural framework, in addition to bone.

How do we overcome this tough collagen, so our penis can grow to its maximum potential?

We break the bonds within the collagen.

Penis Enlargement Like Building a Brick Wall:

Imagine you have a brick wall in front of you. To make it taller, instead of simply adding another row of bricks on top, you suspend the top portion of the brick wall, take out a line of mortar from the center of wall, and then insert another row of bricks. You now have a taller brick wall.

This is what we do to the collagen in the penis, when we do penis enlargement. We break the bonds of collagen, then the collagen rebuilds itself longer than before. Through mitosis, the other tissue in the penis also rebuilds, and the peripheral nerves elongate, making your whole package bigger!

For men new to penis enlargement, you may see some easy first gains due to the nature of the collagen within the penis. Your penis naturally has some crimps or slack in it, if you've never done penis exercises before. When you start your penis exercising routine, these crimps are removed, giving you some fairly quick gains. It's not until the critical traction is applied that the collagen bonds are broken and real enlargement begins.

Ligaments, Skeletal Muscles and Penis Enlargement:

Ligaments also have an effect on your success with penis enlargement. These too are made of collagen fibers and are again relatively inelastic, prohibiting enlargement growth. Like the collagen in the chambers of the penis, the collagen in the ligaments naturally has crimps in it that will straighten out and lengthen, early in the penis exercising process. After that, then the molecular bond breaking and remodeling of the ligaments is what needs to happen to lengthen the ligaments permanently.

The skeletal muscles that serve as attachment points at the base of your penis also affect your penis enlargement results. When you apply traction to the penis, these skeletal muscles undergo hypertrophy, which allows them to then strengthen and allow for enlargement. Think of it similarly as when you do arm curls, and your biceps and triceps get bigger and stronger.

Only by breaking the collagen bonds, so they rebuild longer, and lengthening the other tissues, can you get the penis enlargement results you want.[8]

Appendix C:

Exercise Guide & Advanced Exercises

Exercise Category	Exercise	Intensity Level	Min. Months of Total Exercising Before Use	Found on Page Number
KEGEL	Kegel Start/Stop	1	0	60
	Kegel	1	0	61
	Kegel Slam	1	0	61
	Kegel Endurance	2	1	217
	Penis Raise	2	1	218
	Towel Raise	2	1	219
JELQ	Jelq	1	0	83
	Side Jelq	3	2-3	221
	Vertical Jelq	3	2-3	222
LENGTH	Basic Stretch	1	0	90
	JAI Stretch	1	0	94
	Rotating Stretch	2	1	224
	Pendulum Stretch	2	1	225
	Internal Stretch	3	2-3	226
	Twisting Stretch	3	2-3	227
	Double Stretch	3	2-3	228
	BTC Stretch	4	3-4	229
	A-Stretch	4	3-4	230
	V-Stretch	4	3-4	231
	Double Rotating	5	4-6	232

Exercise Category	Exercise	Intensity Level	Min. Months of Total Exercising Before Use	Found on Page Number
Girth	Squeeze	2	1	234
	Flaccid Bend	2	1	235
	Side Jelq	3	2-3	221
	Vertical Jelq	3	2-3	222
	Uli	4	3-4	236
	Double Uli	4	3-4	237
	Backwards Uli Jelq	5	4-6	238
	Jelqing Uli	5	4-6	239
	Headhold Jelq	5	4-6	240
	Slinky Bend	5	4-6	241
	Horse Squeeze	5	4-6	242
CIRCUITS	Length Circuit	5	4-6	244
	Girth Circuit	6	6-9	245
CURVE	Straight Stretch	1	0	90/178
	Mini Jelq	1	0	179
	Straight Bend: Flaccid	2	1	179/235
	Side Jelq, Vertical Jelq	3	2-3	221/222
	Straight Bend: Slinky	5	4-6	179/241

Key Notes for Exercise Descriptions

Erection Level:

The *"erection gauge"* is on page 78.

Recommended Reps:

Each exercise has a recommended number of reps. You should stick with this number for the first week or two of using a new exercise. Thereafter, you can gradually increase the number of reps as long as you have healthy body clues.

Lubrication:

You will not need to use lubrication unless the exercise instructs it. It is, however, easier on your skin if you use lubrication for all the exercises that involve jelqing, such as the side jelq and the jelqing uli.

Videos:

To help serve as a visual aide, you can find videos of the exercises at http://www.PEGym.com/penis-exercises.

ADVANCED EXERCISE

Kegel Exercises

In this part you will learn:

- The Kegel Endurance
- The Penis Raise
- The Towel Raise

Kegel Endurance

Intensity Level 2: Do Not Use for at Least 1 Month

Recommended Reps: 3

The Exercise:

Kegel and hold the contraction for as long as possible. The goal is to tightly hold the contraction for at least thirty seconds to one minute.

Penis Raise

Intensity Level 2: Do Not Use for at Least 1 Month

The Exercise

Erection Level: 100 percent
Recommended Reps: 30
Steps:

1. While erect, do a kegel. *Your penis should rise.*
2. Push down on your penis while holding the kegel.

Start

Tips!

- *Increase the intensity by holding the kegel contraction for several seconds or more.*

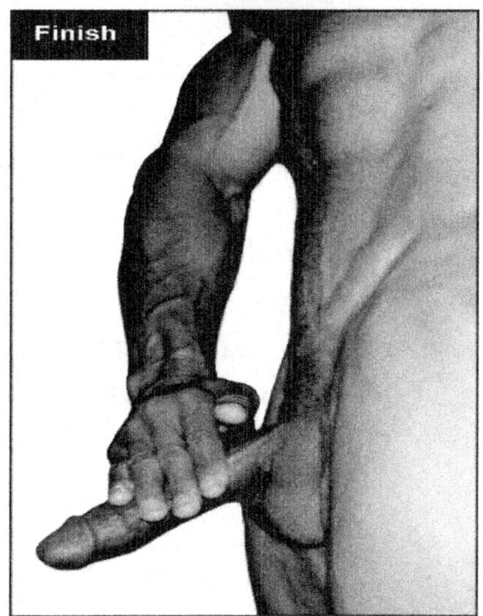

Towel Raise

Intensity Level 2: Do Not Use for at Least 1 Month

The Exercise

Erection Level: 100 percent
Recommended Reps: 30
Steps:

- Place a hand towel on your erect penis.
- Kegel to lift the towel up.

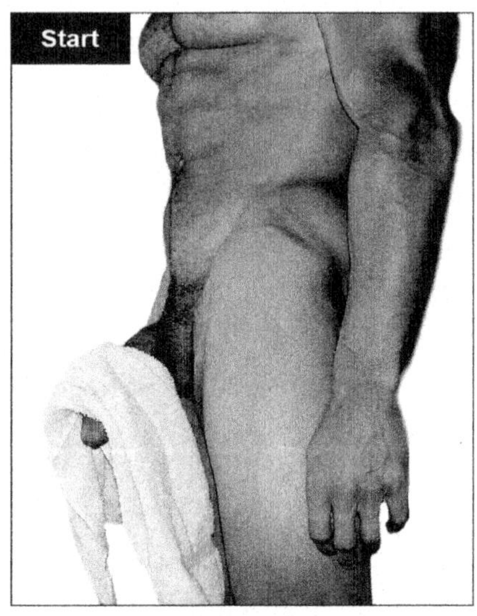

Tips!

- *When your erection starts to subside, place two fingers underneath the penis and squeeze in a few more reps.*
- *At first use a dry hand towel. As you advance, wet the towel for more weight.*

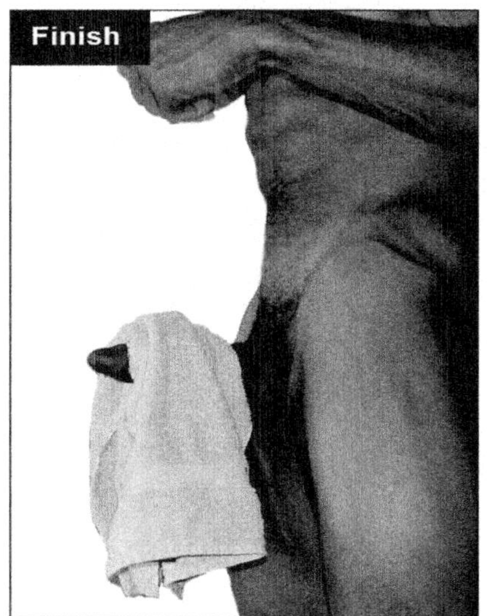

Jelq Exercises

In this part you will learn:

- The Jelq Variation 1: Side Jelq
- The Jelq Variation 2: Vertical Jelq

Jelq Variation 1: Side Jelq

Intensity Level 3: Do Not Use for at Least 2 to 3 Months

The Exercise

Erection Level: 75 to 85 percent

Recommended Reps: 30

Steps:

- Start a normal jelq. At the halfway point, place your other hand at the base of your penis to help build support.
- Simultaneously, curve the jelq to the side. Once you reach the head of your penis, press the palm of your hand against your penis to finish the bending motion. *The entire jelq should last three to five seconds.*
- Repeat in the opposite direction with your other hand.

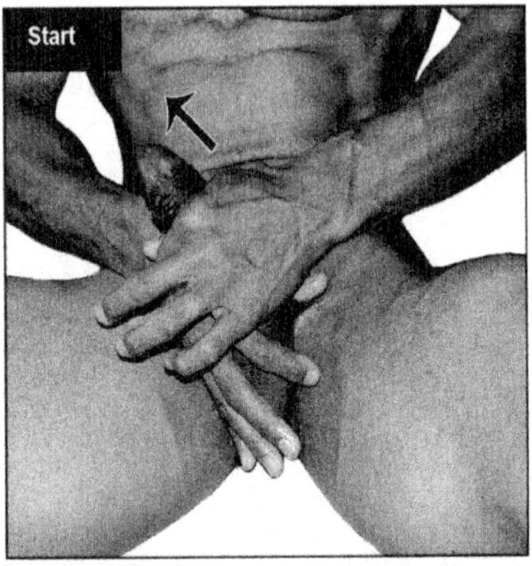

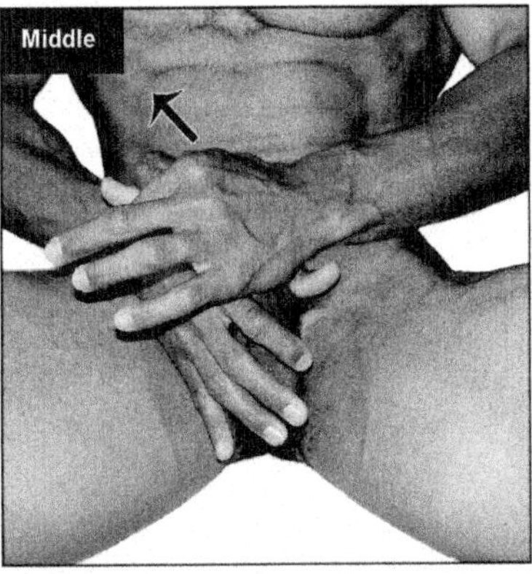

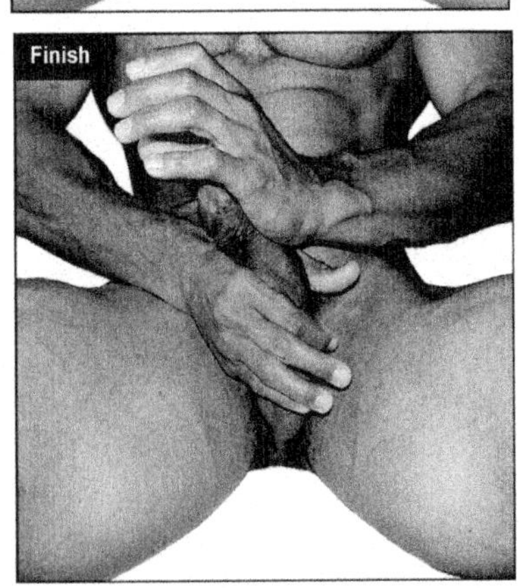

Jelq Variation 2: Vertical Jelq

Intensity Level 3: Do Not Use for at Least 2 to 3 Months

The Exercise

Erection Level: 75 to 85 percent

Recommended Reps: 30

Steps:

- Start a normal jelq.
- At the halfway point, place your other hand at the base of your penis to help build support.
- Towards the end of the jelq, bend the penis downwards in a jelqing motion. *The entire jelq should last three to five seconds.*
- Repeat with your other hand.

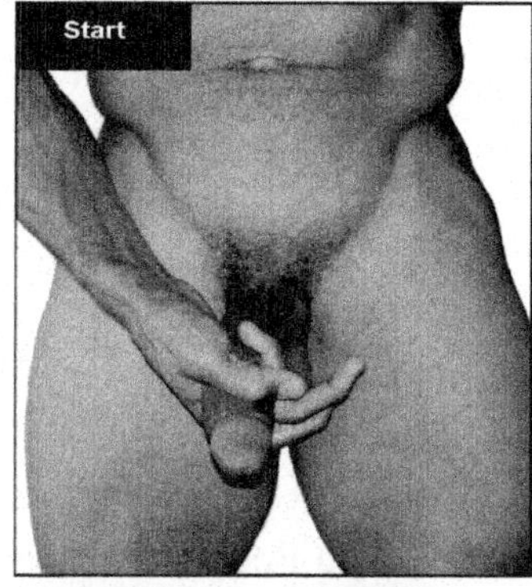

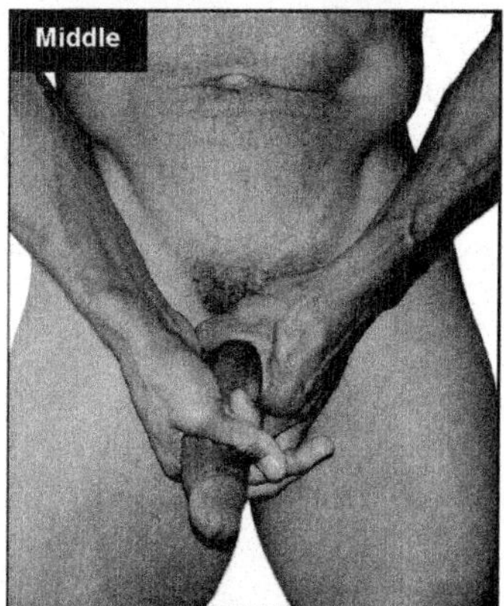

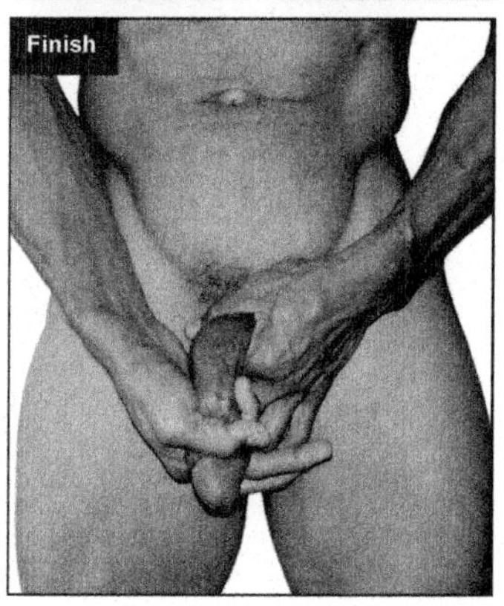

Length Exercises

In this part you will learn:

- The Rotating Stretch
- The Pendulum Stretch
- The Internal Stretch
- The Twisting Stretch
- The Double Stretch
- The BTC (Between the Cheeks) Stretch
- The A-Stretch
- The V-Stretch
- The Double Rotating Stretch

Rotating Stretch

Intensity Level 2: Do Not Use for at Least 1 Month

The Exercise

Erection Level: 0 to 50 percent
Recommended Reps: 10
Steps:

- Stretch your penis straight up.
- In one complete motion, move the stretch to the left; then straight down; then to the right; and then back up again—making a complete circle. The 360 degree stretch should last approximately 10 to 15 seconds.

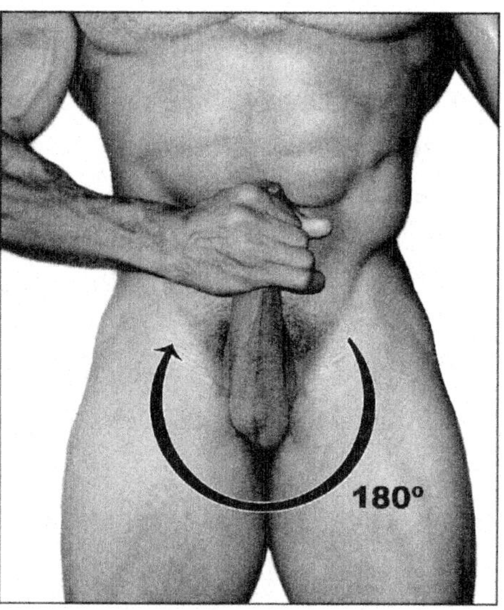

Pendulum Stretch

Intensity Level 2: Do Not Use for at Least 1 Month

The Exercise

Erection Level: 50 percent
Recommended Reps: 50
Steps:

- Stretch your penis down and to the right. Hold one second.
- Now move the stretch down and to the left. Hold one second.

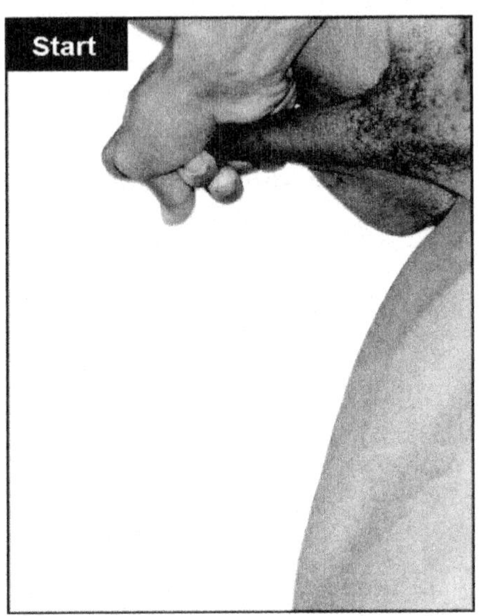

Tips!

- *Do the pendulum stretch at multiple angles—down, straight out, and up.*
- *Continually repeat steps 1 and 2 (in a back and forth pendulum motion).*

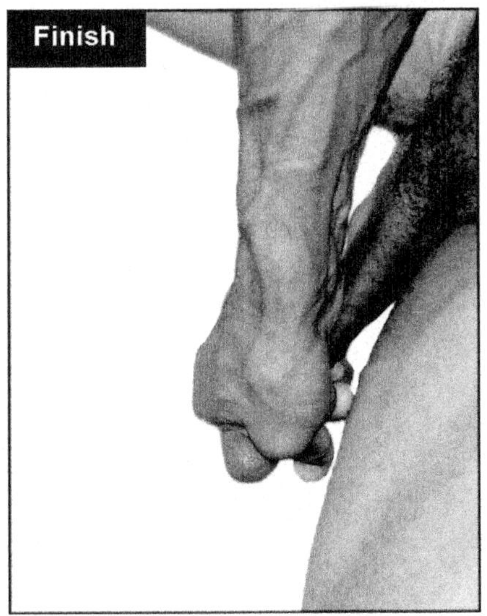

Internal Stretch

Intensity Level 3: Do Not Use for at Least 2 to 3 Months

The Exercise

Erection Level: 0 to 50 percent
Recommended Reps: 5
Steps: This exercise uses two hands.

- Hand 1: Place an OK-grip around the base of your penis and your scrotum. Don't grip the actual testicles.
- Hand 1: Stretch your penis and scrotum towards your body while pulling in an upward direction.
- Hand 2: Simultaneously grip your penis and pull straight up. Hold both hands in place for 20 to 30 seconds.

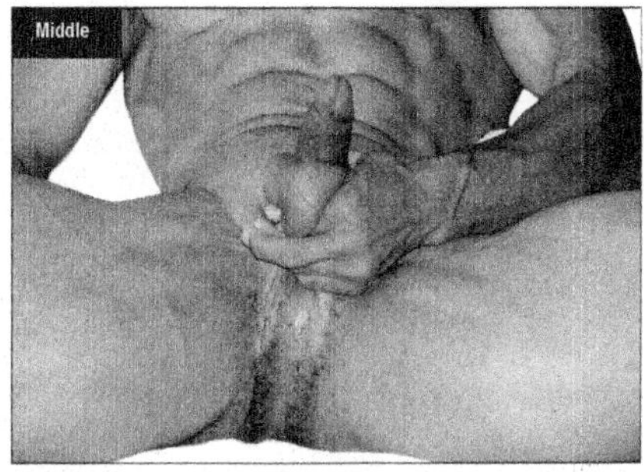

Tips!

- *To increase the intensity, pull up with more force on the hand holding the base of your penis and scrotum.*
- *With this exercise, you'll need to sit down and spread your legs apart.*

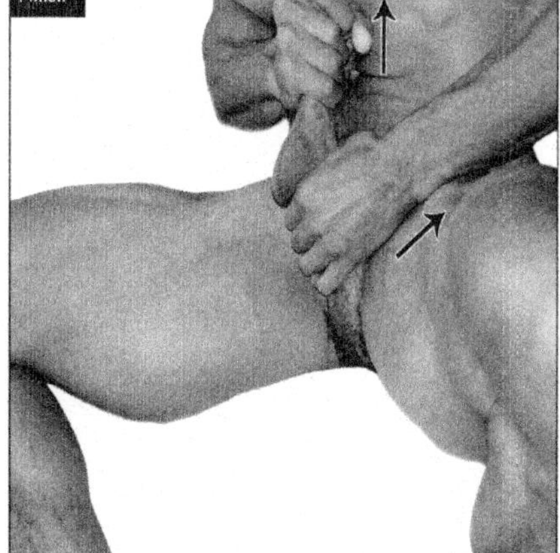

Twisting Stretch

Intensity Level 3: Do Not Use for at Least 2 to 3 Months

The Exercise

Erection Level: 50 percent
Recommended Reps: 5
Steps:

- Twist your penis one to two times, like a screw.
- Simultaneously pull outwards. *Hold for 20 to 30 seconds.*

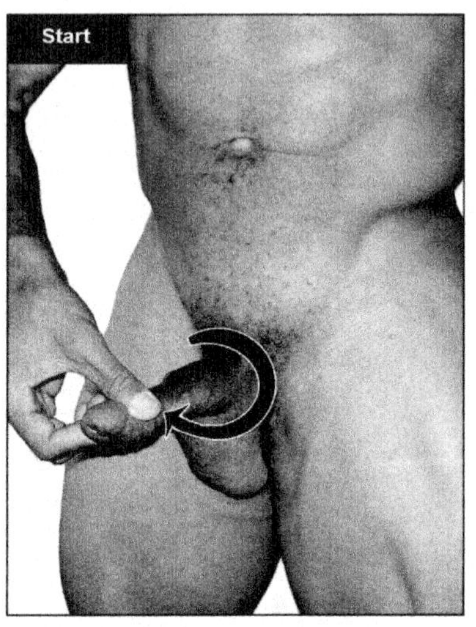

Tips!

- *Continually rotate the direction in which you twist. If you twist to the left one time, twist to the right the next.*

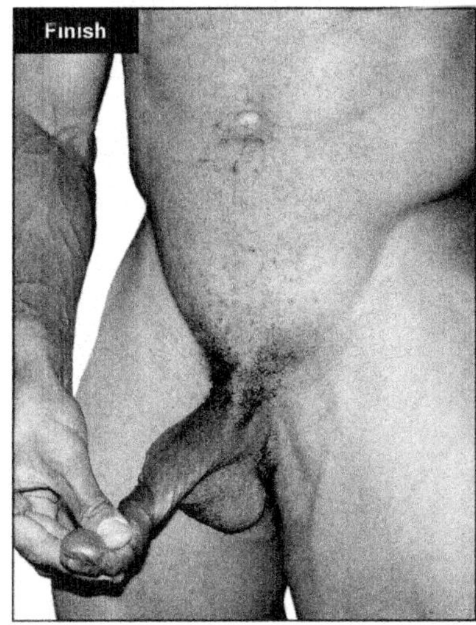

Double Stretch

Intensity Level 3: Do Not Use for at Least 2 to 3 Months

The Exercise

Erection Level: 0 to 50 percent
Recommended Reps: 5
Steps: This exercise uses two hands.

- Hand 1: Grip the penis an inch below the head and pull straight out.
- Hand 2: Grip an inch above the base and pull towards you. At this point you are stretching in two different directions (hand 1 is pulling away from your body; hand 2 is pulling towards your body). *Hold for 20 to 30 seconds.*

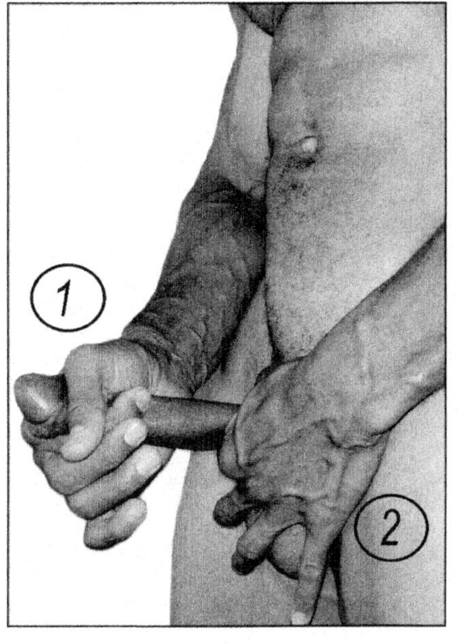

Tips!

- *Constantly change up the points where you grip to give your entire penis a complete workout.*

-Between the Cheeks Stretch (BTC)-

Intensity Level 4: Do Not Use for at Least 3 to 4 Months

The Exercise

Erection Level: 0 to 50 percent
Recommended Reps: 5
Steps:

- Stand with your leg propped up on a chair, a toilet seat, or anything knee-level.
- Reach your arm behind your back and grip your penis between your legs. *As always, don't directly grip the head of your penis.*
- Pull your penis between your legs and upwards. Your penis should be stretched behind you, between your cheeks. *Hold the stretch for 20 to 30 seconds.*

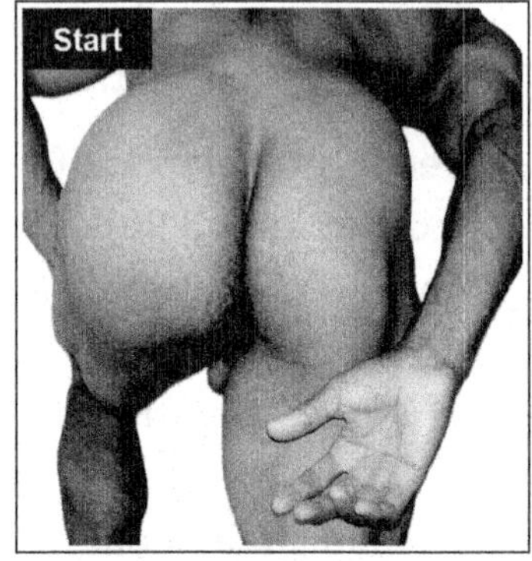

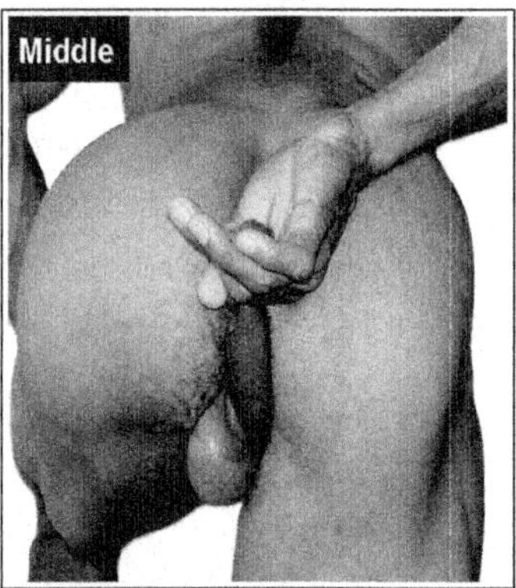

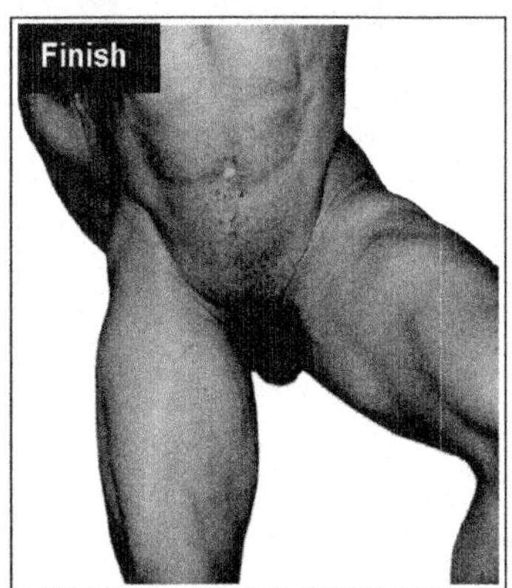

A-Stretch

Intensity Level 4: Do Not Use for at Least 3 to 4 Months

The Exercise

Erection Level: 0 to 50 percent
Recommended Reps: 5
Steps: This exercise uses two hands.

- Hand 1: Grip the penis an inch below the head and pull straight out.
- Hand 2: Place your arm underneath the stretched penis.
- Hand 2: Push upwards with your entire arm, using it as a lever. Hold for 20 to 30 seconds.

Tips!

- *The more force you use to push up with the arm underneath the penis, the more intense the stretch.*
- *For even more intensity, use hand 2 (the hand underneath the penis) to grip the wrist of hand 1 (the wrist holding the stretch).*

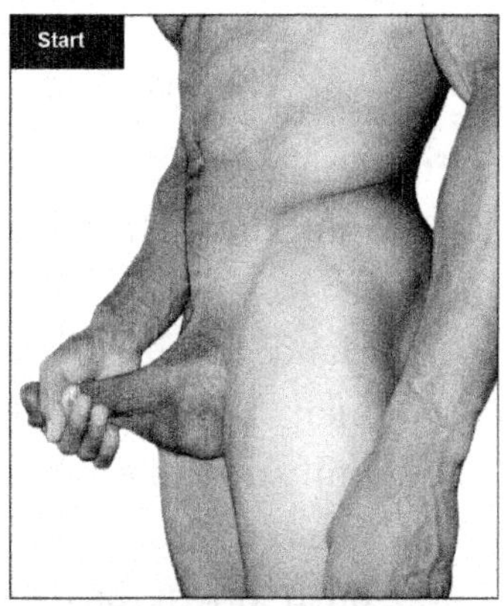
Start

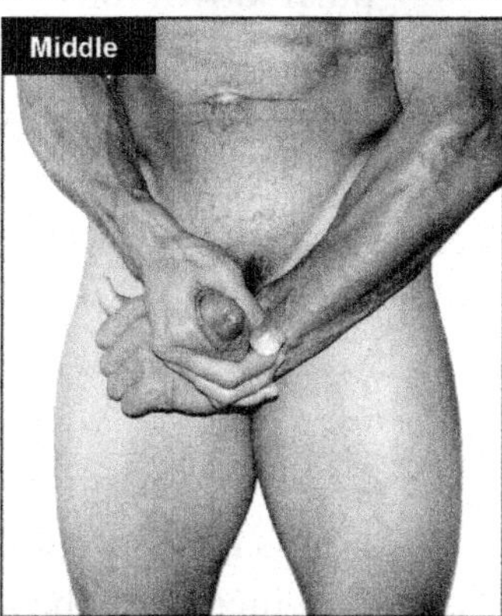
Middle

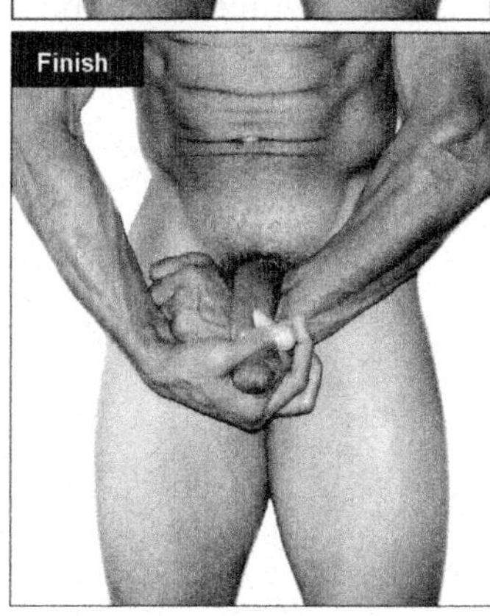
Finish

V-Stretch

Intensity Level 4: Do Not Use for at Least 3 to 4 Months

The Exercise

Erection Level: 50 percent
Recommended Reps: 5
Steps:

- Hand 1: Grip the penis an inch below the head and pull straight out.
- Hand 2: Use your thumb to push down on your penis. Hold both the stretch and the downward push for 20 to 30 seconds.

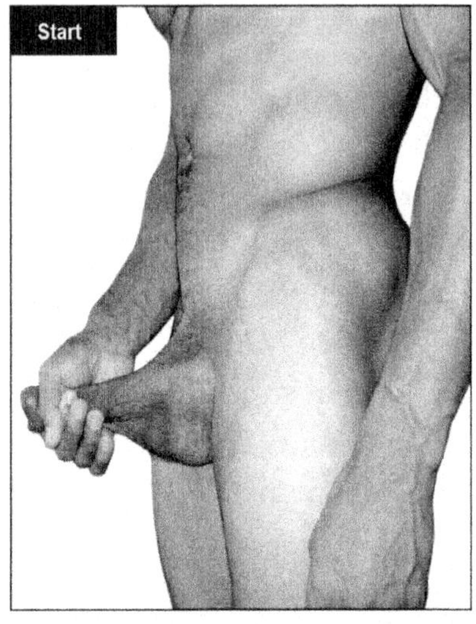

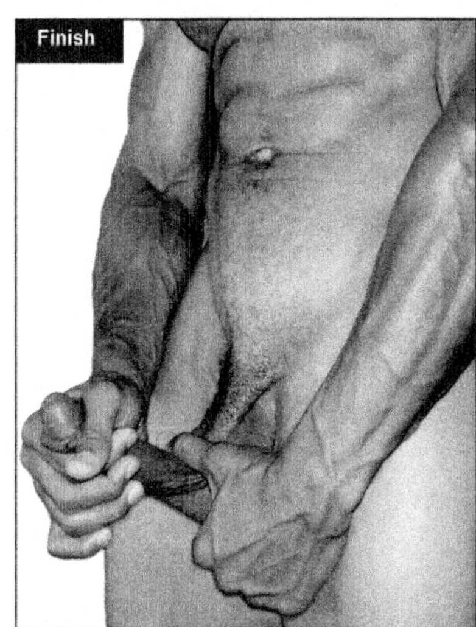

Tips!

- Press down on different points of your shaft.
- To increase the intensity, use your wrist to push downwards.

Double Rotating Stretch

Intensity Level 5: Do Not Use for at Least 4 to 6 Months

The Exercise

Erection Level: 0 to 50 percent
Recommended Reps: 10
Steps: This exercise uses two hands.

- Hand 1: Grip your penis an inch below the head and pull straight up.
- Hand 2: Grip the penis an inch above the base and pull towards your testes.
- Hand 1: Slowly stretch your penis in a single circular motion. Move the stretch to the left; then straight down; then to the right; and then back up again—making a complete circle. *The circular rotation should last approximately 10 to 15 seconds.*

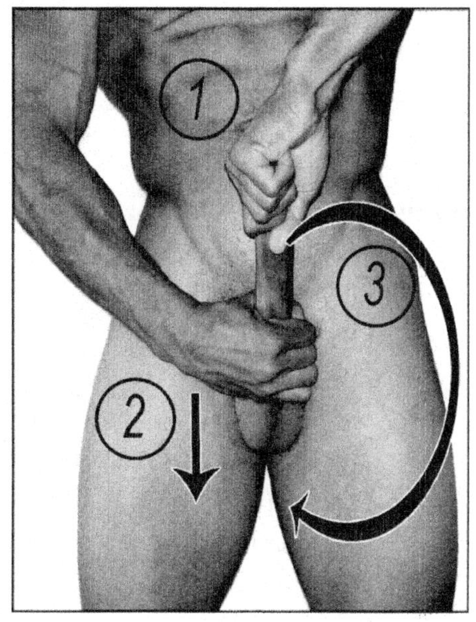

Finish Girth Exercises

In this part you will learn:

- The Squeeze
- The Flaccid Bend
- The ULI
- The ULI Variation 1: Double ULI
- The ULI Variation 2: Backwards ULI Jelq
- The ULI Variation 3: Jelqing ULI
- The Headhold Jelq
- The Slinky Bend
- The Horse Squeeze

Squeeze

Intensity Level 2: Do Not Use for at Least 1 Month

The Exercise

Erection Level: 50 to 75 percent

Recommended Reps: 5

Steps: This exercise uses two hands.

- Hand 1: Form a tight OK-grip as close to the base as possible.
- Hand 2: In front of the first grip, form an overhand OK-grip—with your fingers facing the floor.
- Both Hands: Tighten all of your fingers and squeeze both grips. *Hold for 20 to 30 seconds.*

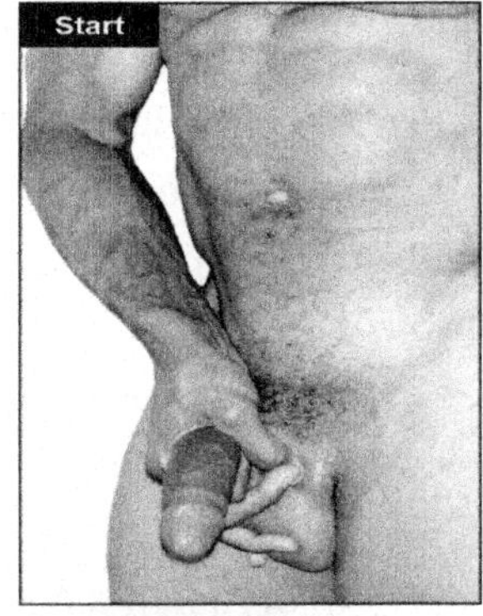

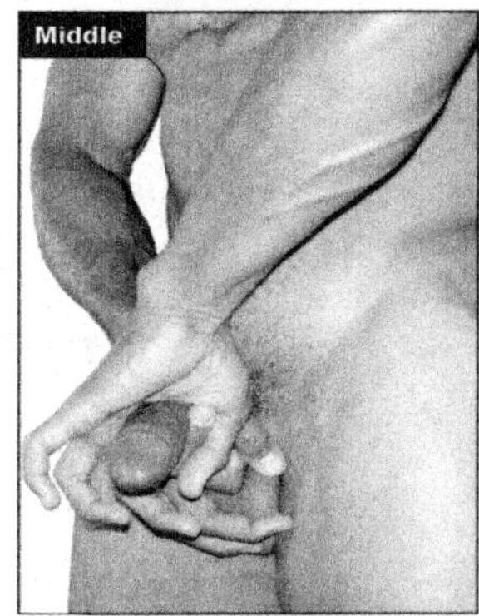

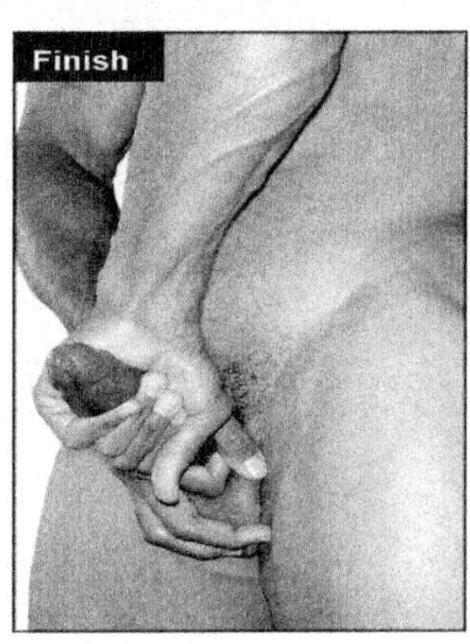

Tips!

- *For increased intensity, kegel to push more blood into the penis.*

Flaccid Bend

Intensity Level 2: Do Not Use for at Least 1 Month

The Exercise

Erection Level: 25 to 50 percent
Recommended Reps: 5
Steps: This exercise uses two hands.

- Hand 1: Grip the penis below the head of your penis, as if you were going to stretch.
- Hand 2: Place two to four fingers underneath the penis.
- Hand 1: Bend the penis over the fingers. *Hold for 20 to 30 seconds.*

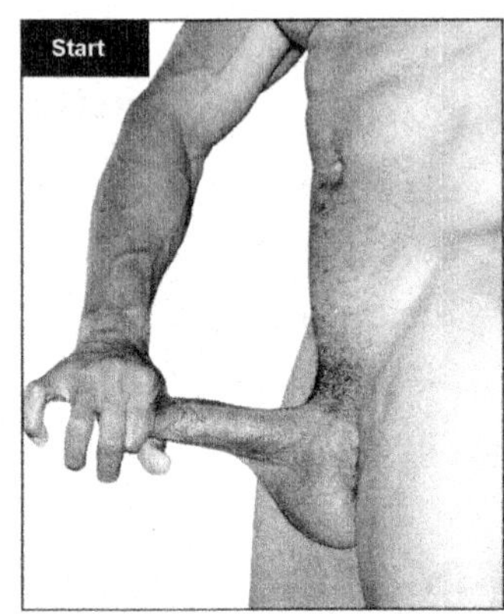

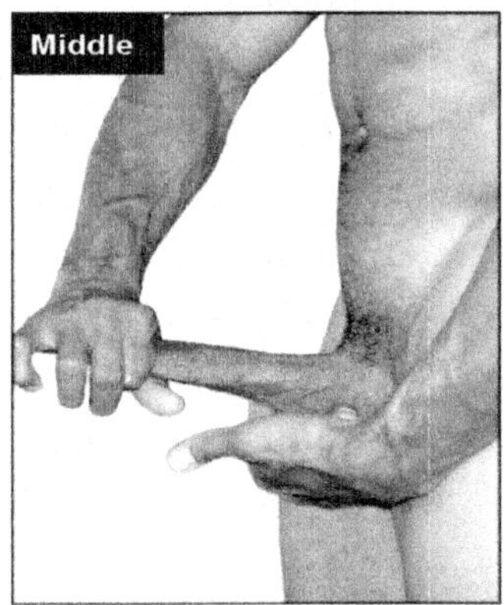

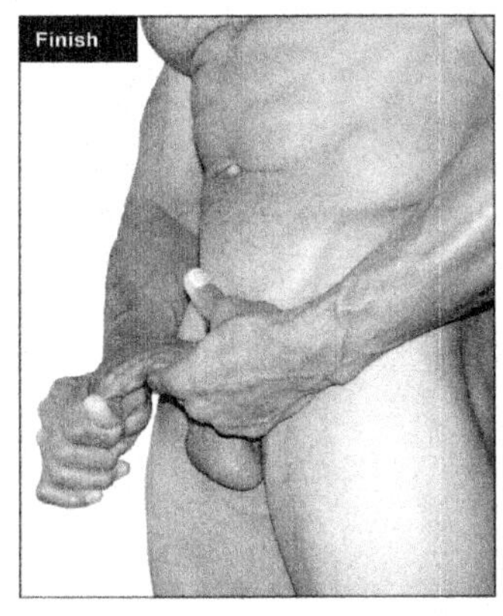

Tips!

- *Do an entire flaccid bend workout by repeating steps one through three in each direction. Do this by placing the fingers above the shaft to bend up; to the right of the shaft to bend right; and to the left of the shaft to bend left.*
- *As time goes on, increase the intensity by repeating the exercise several times. But each time place a different number of fingers underneath the penis.*

ULI

Intensity Level 4: Do Not Use for at Least 3 to 4 Months

The Exercise

Erection Level: 100 percent
Recommended Reps: 3
Steps:

- Form a grip at the base of your penis. You can either use an OK-grip or your entire hand.
- Squeeze the grip tightly. Hold for 30 to 60 seconds.

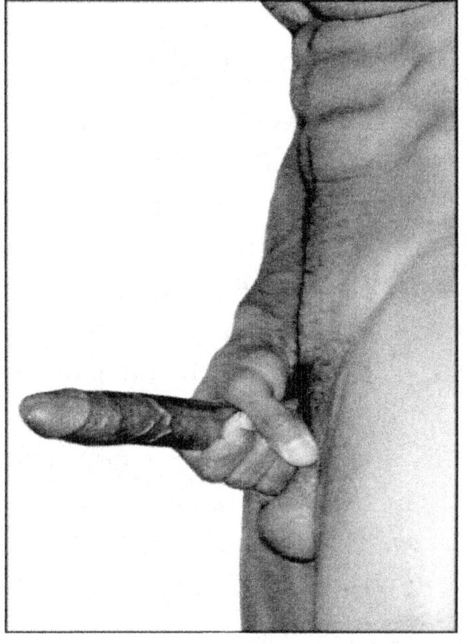

Tips!

- *Position the grip as close to the base as possible so you can fill your entire penis with blood.*

ULI Variation 1: Double ULI

Intensity Level 4: Do Not Use for at Least 3 to 4 Months

The Exercise

Erection Level: 100 percent
Recommended Reps: 3
Steps: This exercise uses two hands.

- Hand 1: Form a grip at the base of your penis.
- Kegel more blood into the penis.
- Hand 2: Form a grip right below the head.
- Tightly squeeze both grips. Hold for thirty to sixty seconds.

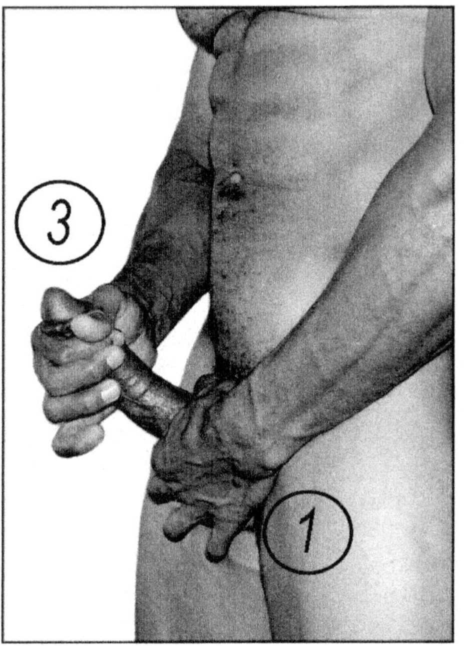

Finish ULI Variation 2: Backwards ULI Jelq

Intensity Level 5: Do Not Use for at Least 4 to 6 Months

The Exercise

Erection Level: 90 to 95 percent
Recommended Reps: 30
Steps: This exercise uses two hands.

- Hand 1: Form a tight OK-grip at the base of your erect penis.
- Hand 2: Place another OK-grip right below the head.
- Hand 2: Do 30 jelqs (the recommended reps) in a backwards motion, pushing the blood towards the base grip. *Each backwards jelq should last approximately 3 to 5 seconds.*

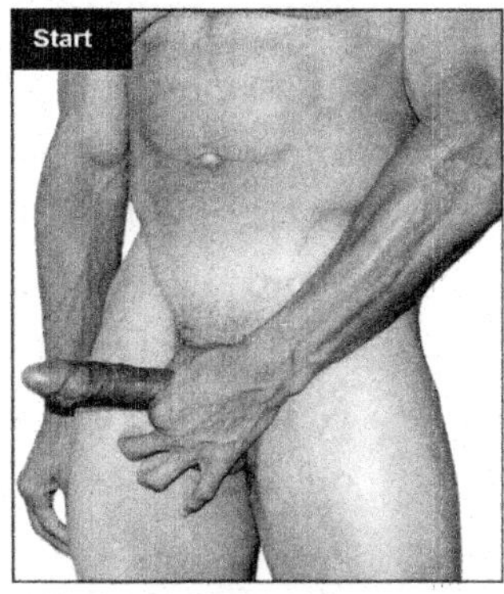

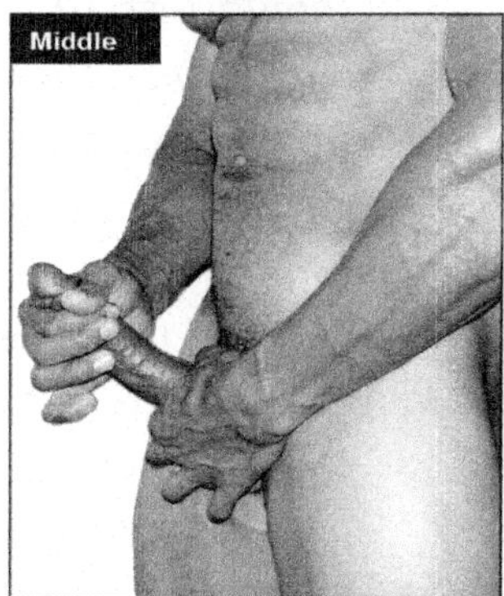

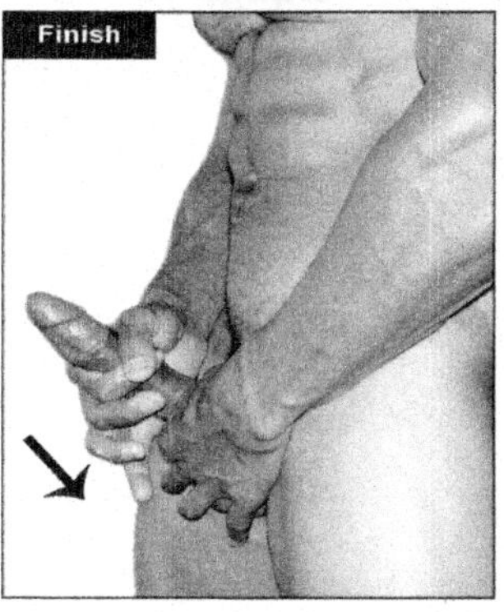

ULI Variation 3: Jelqing ULI

Intensity Level 5: Do Not Use for at Least 4 to 6 Months

The Exercise

Erection Level: 90 to 95 percent
Recommended Reps: 10
Steps: This exercise uses two hands.

- Hand 1: Form a tight OK-grip at the base of your erect penis.
- Hand 2: Form a second OK-grip on top of the first one and slowly jelq it up the penis. *The jelq should last 10 to 15 seconds. You have completed one rep.*
- Immediately after the slow jelq, switch hands so that hand 2 is formed into a tight OK-grip at the base of the penis, and hand 1 is slowly jelqing the penis.
- Continually alternate between hand 1 and hand 2, with one hand jelqing your penis slowly and the other hand maintaining the OK-grip.

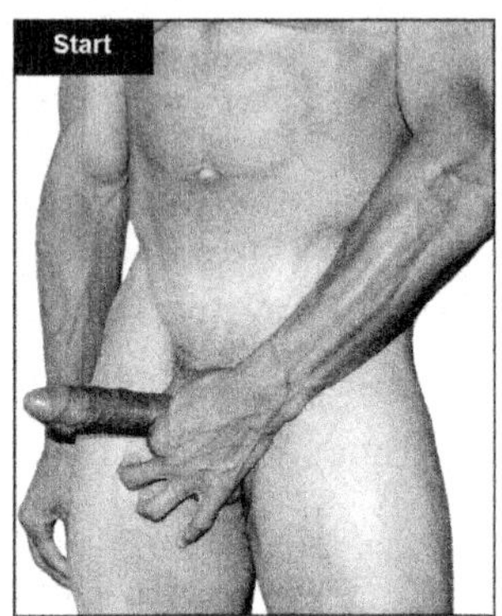

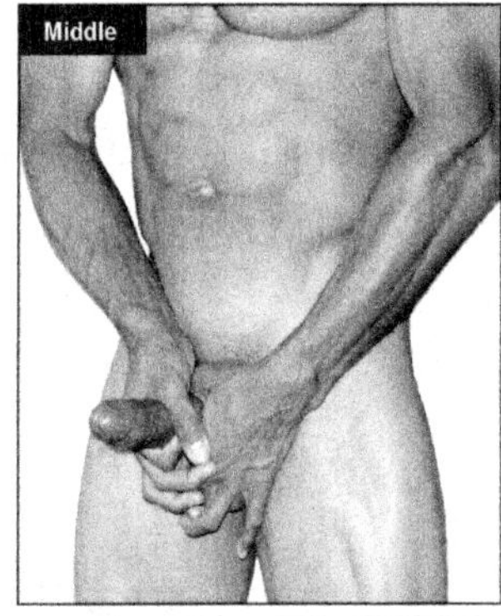

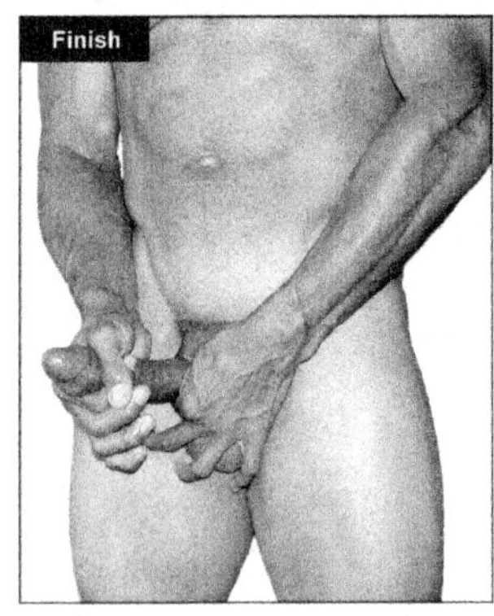

Tips!

- *Keep a tight OK-grip around the base of the penis at all times.*

Headhold Jelq

Intensity Level 5: Do Not Use for at Least 4 to 6 Months

The Exercise

Erection Level: 90 to 95 percent

Recommended Reps: 1

Steps: This exercise uses two hands.

- Hand 1: Form a tight OK-grip at the base of your penis and perform a slow jelq.
- Hand 1: Stop the jelq right below the head, tightly squeeze the grip, and kegel. Keep the grip in place.
- Hand 2: Do thirty jelqs, pushing the blood in the penis towards the head grip. *Each jelq should last 3 to 5 seconds.*

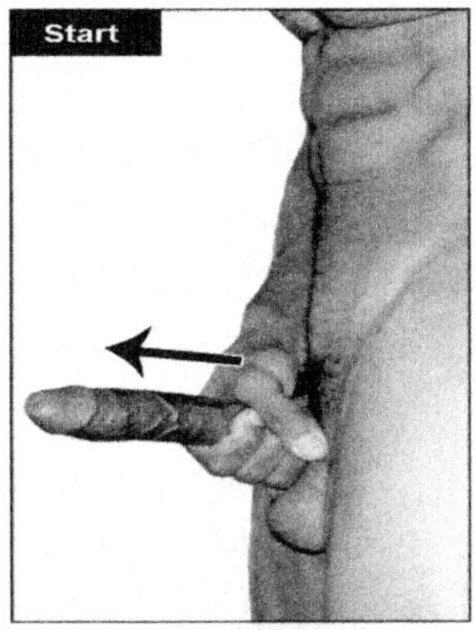

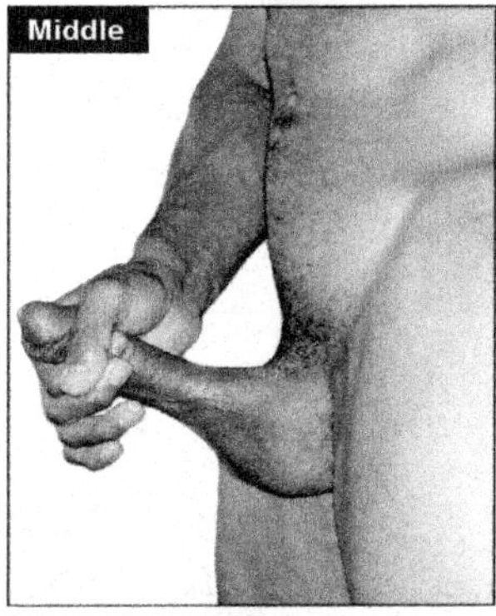

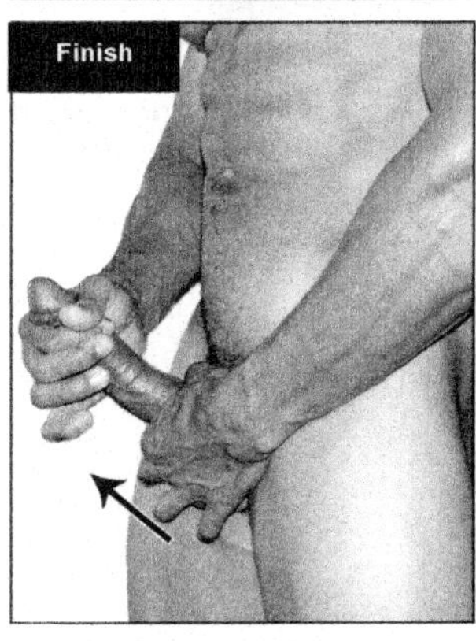

Tips!

- *During the exercise, continually kegel to push more blood into the penis.*

Slinky Bend

Intensity Level 5: Do Not Use for at Least 4 to 6 Months

The Exercise

Erection Level: 80 percent
Recommended Reps: 30
Steps: This exercise uses two hands.

- Hand 1: Form an OK-grip at the base of your penis.
- Hand 2: Form an overhand grip right below the head.
- Hand 2: Slightly bend the penis downwards.
- Push the bend upwards and release.

Tips!

- *The entire bend should take roughly 3 to 5 seconds.*
- *Do the slinky in all four directions: down, up, left, and right.*

Start

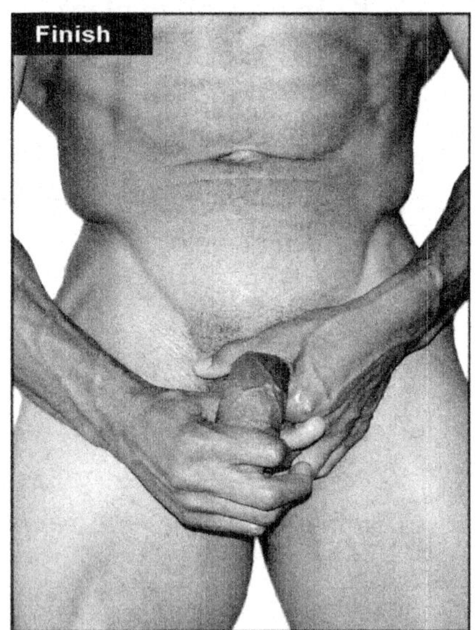

Horse Squeeze

Intensity Level 5: Do Not Use for at Least 4 to 6 Months

The Exercise

Erection Level: 95 percent
Recommended Reps: 6
Steps: This exercise uses two hands. Your penis will need to be lubricated.

- Hand 1: Form a tight OK-grip at the base of your penis.
- Hand 2: Form a small overhand OK-grip, roughly the size of a dime.
- Hand 2: Slowly slide the grip over the head and towards the base of your penis. *It should take roughly 20 seconds for you to get to the base hand.*

Tips!

- *Once your second hand reaches the base hand, increase the intensity by doing the "squeeze" exercise at the base for an additional 30 seconds.*

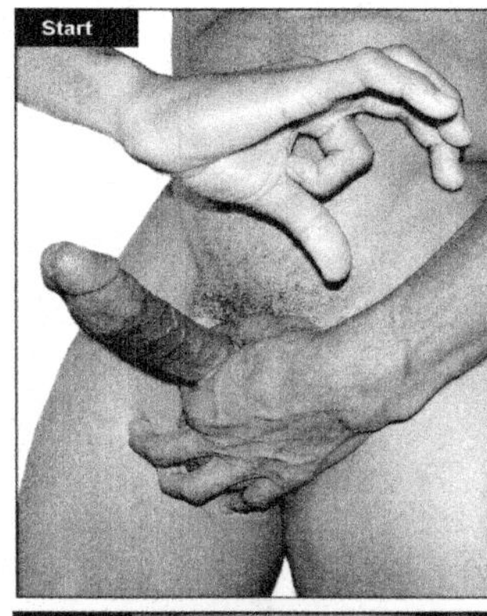

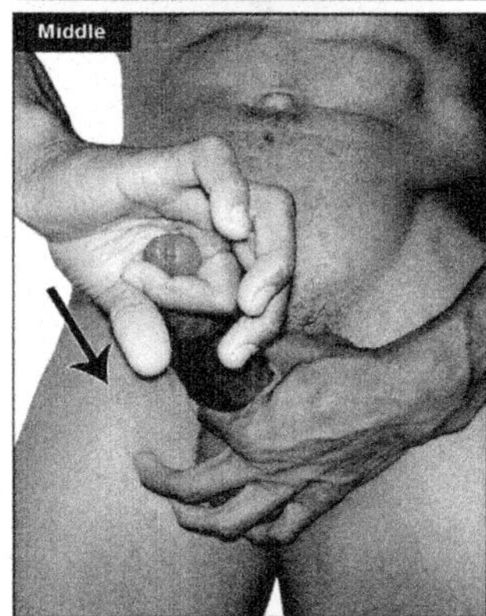

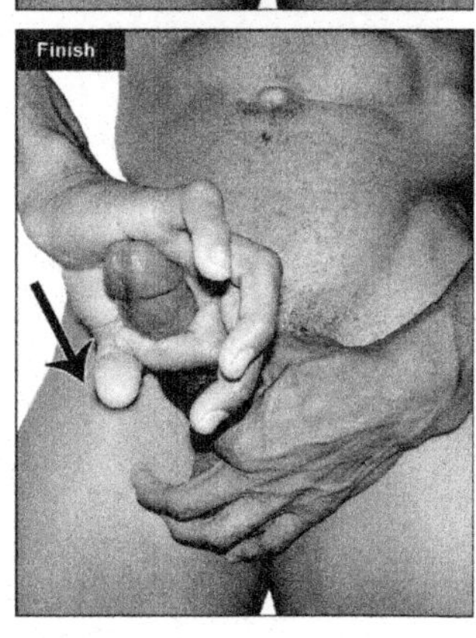

Circuit Exercises

In this part you will learn:

- The Length Circuit
- The Girth Circuit

Length Circuit

Intensity Level 5: Do Not Use for at Least 4 to 6 Months

Here is an example of a length circuit (in which you do several stretches with no rest in between). You can mix and match the exercises. In the beginning, only do the circuit once. Overtime, repeat the circuit and add more exercises to increase the intensity. As an added tip, it helps if you Kegel throughout the circuit.

Do the following exercises one right after the other:

Step	Exercise	Time Frame
1	50 **JAI Stretches**	~1 to 2 minutes
2	5 **Rotating Stretches**	~1 minute
3	10 **A-Stretches**	~4 minutes
4	10 **Double Rotating Stretches**	~2 minutes
5	1 set of the **Basic Stretch**	~2 to 3 minute

Girth Circuit

Intensity Level 6: Do Not Use for at Least 6 to 9 Months

Here is an example of a girth circuit. You can mix and match the exercises. The first few times, only do the circuit once. Thereafter, gradually move up to repeating the entire process for a total of 30 to 45 minutes. You can make the circuit less intense by replacing the *slinkys and jelqing ulis* with *flaccid bends*. Similarly, you can increase the intensity by adding more exercises.

When it comes to girth circuits, you'll get the best workout if you throw masturbation into the mix. That's because right before you ejaculate (at the point of no return), your penis is completely full of blood, and the tissues are expanded to the peak of their normal limit. As an added tip, it helps if you Kegel throughout the circuit.

Do the following exercises one right after the other:

Step	Exercise	Time Frame
1	Do **any stretch.** This will prepare your tissues to expand outward.	~1 to 2 minutes
2	**Masturbate** until you get close to *the point of no return* (don't ejaculate).	As long as it takes
3	Do 1 **Uli**	~1 minute
4	Do 5 **Jelqing Ulis**	~1 minute
5	At this point, your erection level should be below 90. Do 10 *slow* **Jelqs.**	~1 minute
6	Do 20 **Slinkys**	~1 minute
7	Do 1 long **Squeeze**	~1 minute

Appendix D:

Penis Exercising Resources

This resource guide will help you find ways to enhance your penis exercises routine. Here you will find a progress journal sheet, the ingredients for Essential Vein Oil, a selective directory of the best free websites relating to penis exercises, and the average gains-time assessment for the men who took place in my penis exercises survey.

Progress Journal

Copy the progress journal on the following page and put several copies in a binder. Record your workouts to help you track your progress. You can also find the progress journal page online at http://www.PEGym.com/progress.

Progress Journal Sheet

Starting Size:	Current Size:	Goal Size:
L ______ G ________	L ________ G ________	L ________ G ________

Exercise	Intensity of Workout	Time/Reps
	Low/Med/High	

Days Exercised This Week (circle): M T W T F S S

EVO: Essential Vein Oil

Choosing a proper lubricant is important. A good lubricant encourages healthy, flexible skin. A bad lubricant causes skin to go dry and chafe. At first, any of the popular lubricants will most likely suffice. As time goes on, you may want an extra kick in your lubricant. Essential Vein Oil is just that.

EVO was originally created by a penis exerciser name Eroset to help with a minor penis exercises injury—most likely penile Mondor's disease. EVO dissipated Eroset's problem in just a few days. Many men have had similar success with EVO. The lubricant is also great for hardness as it increases blood flow to the penis. Below are the ingredients and instructions for making EVO, directly from the creator himself.[10]

Ingredients

You should be able to find these ingredients in most natural health stores. Make sure that you are buying Pure Essential Oils (NOT fragrance oils or scented oils—both are harsh on the skin):

- **1 cup of Extra Virgin Olive Oil** as a base carrier for the essential oils. Men with sensitive skin will want to use more than a cup of olive oil to dilute the essential oils. To be safe, use at least a cup at first. You may eventually use less olive oil, but it is suggested that you do it slowly.
- **6 ml of Lavender Essential Oil** (organic or 40/42 oil).
- **2.5 ml of Rosemary Essential Oil.** Men with sensitive skin will want to go easy on this and may want to use less than the 2.5 mL suggestion. If you experience unpleasant irritation, this is the oil to look at first. Rosemary is the best vasodilator in the mix and great penetrating oil, but it's also the harshest on the skin.
- **2 ml of Clary Sage Essential Oil.**
- **1.5-2 ml of Lemongrass Essential Oil**. Men with sensitive skin will want to go easy on this as well.

Instructions

Pour the oils into a bottle and shake to ensure the oils are mixed. Do this before every use. If you are using EVO for the first time, you must test it on something other than your penis first. Test EVO by placing a tiny bit on a cotton swab and apply it to the inside of your wrist or your inner elbow. Don't wash the area for twenty-four hours. If no redness or itching occurs, then the EVO should be safe to use. Even still, use just a tiny amount the first time. If itching or redness does occur, add another cup of extra virgin olive oil to dilute the essential oils, and try again.

Essential oils are potent. Use them with caution if you're a first time user. "When used intelligently, essential oils are far less likely to cause side effects than most over-the-counter drugs," says author Bill Gottlied in New Choices in Natural Healing. "But experts still advice proceeding with caution. In general, people with fair or freckled skin are more likely to experience skin irritation from essential oils."

Depending on the sensitivity of your skin, you might have an allergic reaction to essential oils. Also, keep essential oils away from pregnant women, and avoid using essential oils if you have high blood pressure or epilepsy. For these reasons, you are using essential oils at your own risk.

Your Companion Website

PEGym.com:

The PE Gym is a prime information resource for penis exercises and male sexual health information. It is also the companion for countless readers of this book. On this website, you'll receive free access to:

- An online community where you can ask questions, read the experiences of other penis exercisers, and share your insights with thousands of others.
- Videos of the exercises in this book along with dozens more to help you nail down your technique.
- Hundreds of published penis exercises articles and guides.

- Information on penis health, penis enlargement devices, and popular sex topics such as lasting longer in the bedroom.
- A penis enlargement glossary for the frequently used terms in this book.

Other Great Websites

Altpenis.com:

The website that discusses all aspects of your favorite organ—including the use, abuse, care, and maintenance of it.

Betterman.com:

A male improvement community forum with information on penis exercises, penis enlargement devices, and numerous other mens health issues.

Bibhanger.com/Forums:

A support forum for the popular Bib Hanger, along with information on other penis enlargement methods.

LPSG.org:

The Large Penis Support Group has information on penis exercises and other penis-health related issues, along with the largest community in the world that focuses on how to use and maintain a large penis.

Mattersofsize.com/Forums:

A large penis enlargement forum with over 100,000 registered users and a support forum.

Thundersplace.com:

For nearly ten years now, Thunder's Place has been a leading free information source on penis exercises and penis enlargement. Its premier content is built through its thousands of users, which makes it an unbiased place to learn more about penis enlargement. Thunder's Place is more than just a community though, it also has a free penis enlargement guide (which is rare on the World Wide Web), free penis exercises videos, instructions for building common penis enlargement devices, and more. The active members at Thunder's Place are willing to go above and beyond to help out a fellow penis exerciser—several of whom helped build the knowledge that is provided in this book.

Average Gains-Time Assessment

Here you will find a more detailed assessment on how long it took the men in my survey to make their gains. For this assessment, the men were broken down into four different groups, depending on how much they gained. From there, the men of each individual group were broken down into four more groups, depending on how long they had been performing penis exercises.

You should note that the following results are just what the men reported. As with all surveys, there is bound to be error in what was said and what actually occurred. Moreover, performing penis exercises is still a new "art." There have been great discoveries over the past few years that have lead to men gaining more in a shorter period of time, and there's bound to be more discoveries over the next few years as well.

Length

Out of 207 men who gained between 0.25 and 0.74 inches of length:
69.7% had exercised their penis for 6 months or less
15.3 % exercised between 7 to 12 months
9.2 % exercised between 13 to 24 months
5.3 % exercised between 2 years or more

Out of 150 men who gained <u>between 0.75 and 1.24 inches</u> of length:
38.1 % exercised for 6 months or less
30.7 % exercised between 7 to 12 months
19.3 % exercised between 13 to 24 months
11.9 % exercised between 2 years or more

Out of 104 men who gained <u>between 1.25 and 1.99 inches</u> of length:
28.9 % exercised for 6 months or less
20.2 % exercised between 7 to 12 months
23.1 % exercised between 13 to 24 months
27.9 % exercised between 2 years or more

Out of 57 men who gained <u>2 inches or more</u> of length:
15.9 % exercised for 6 months or less
15.9 % exercised between 7 to 12 months
22.8 % exercised between 13 to 24 months
45.5 % exercised between 2 years or more

Girth

Out of 225 men who gained <u>between 0.1 and 0.49 inches</u> of girth:
59.5 % had exercised their penis for 6 months or less
21.8 % exercised between 7 to 12 months
8.8 % exercised between 13 to 24 months
9.8 % exercised between two years or more

Out of 175 men who gained <u>between 0.5 and 0.99 inches</u> of girth:
38.8 % exercised for 6 months or less
22.8 % exercised between 7 to 12 months
18.8 % exercised between 13 to 24 months
19.3 % exercised between two years or more

Out of 58 men who gained <u>between 1 and 1.49 inches</u> of girth:
17.3 % exercised for 6 months or less
22.4 % exercised between 7 to 12 months

34.5 % exercised between 13 to 24 months
25.8 % exercised between two years or more

Out of 27 men who gained 1.5 inches or more of girth:
29.6 % exercised for 6 months or less
11.1 % exercised between 7 to 12 months
18.5 % exercised between 13 to 24 months
40.7 % exercised between two years or more

Why Not More?

You might notice that the majority of the men gained an inch or less in either length or girth. The reason for this could be that:

1. Some men gain length easily; others gain girth easily. So, for instance, a man who gained only 0.25 inches in length could have gained over an inch in girth.
2. Some men have smaller goals, and don't necessarily want to gain more than a half inch or so.
3. Gains generally become more difficult to obtain as time goes on
4. Motivation decreases overtime for some men, often because they start performing penis exercises due to feeling small; but the more they gain, the less they care about penis size.
5. There is such a thing as too big. Since most men start out average, adding multiple inches might build a penis bigger than many men want, or at least would want to put in the time for.
6. The men could have impeded growth by continually over-training and performing penis exercises improperly.
7. The men might not have been performing penis exercises long enough to see any gains yet, as any man—regardless of how little they had exercised their penis—were allowed to take the survey. Indeed, when only the men who had been performing penis exercises for at least three months were used, the average gain was 1 inch in length and 0.5 inches in girth. Accordingly, not every man who took the survey gained. Out of 684 men who answered the appropriate questions to be a part of the Average Gains-Time Assessment, 617 of them gained in length, girth, or both.[11]

Appendix E:

Penis Exercising Success Stories

The best part about writing this book was the success stories. They were both insightful and motivational.[12] On the following pages, you will find several encouraging success stories. You can find more penis exercises success stories at http://www.PEGym.com/success, where I also look forward to reading your success story one day. Note that in the success stories that follow, the real name used is sometimes a fictitious name. The online alias is the name that the man used in the penis exercises community.

"I Tripled My Penis Size With Just Jelqs and Stretches!"

Name: Gary
Online Alias: Higherone
Age: 32
Starting Size: Length 4.5", Girth 4"
Current Size: Length 7.25", Girth 5.25"

Gary, a teacher in Western Pennsylvania, started performing penis exercises because he wasn't satisfied with his size. "I went to an all boys high school and we had to shower for gym. It was pretty obvious I wasn't packing. Porn didn't help either. It was an eye-opener seeing guys with big dicks and my dick being small."

So Gary did what many other men do when they feel small and inadequate: he avoided sex. After several years of hiding from his size, an online buddy introduced Gary to penis exercises, and he was optimistic. "At the time, I didn't believe it worked as much as I hoped it worked. I would have done anything to get a bigger dick at that point," says Gary. Luckily, "I ended up gaining a quarter inch pretty fast . . . you would have thought I won the lottery!" (He opted not to call his family and friends to tell them the news).

Gary gradually increased the intensity by adding time to his workouts. He stopped adding time to his routine after his workouts reached an hour, but he continued to increase the intensity of his jelqs and stretches. "I gradually used more force and pulled harder," he reports. In roughly a year he gained 1.5 inches in length and nearly an inch in girth—putting him right at the statistical average. Over the next two years, he continued to perform penis exercises on and off and gained enough to put him well above average—and increase his size by nearly 300 percent.

At one point, Gary's brother caught him performing penis exercises. Gary had no choice but to spill the beans to his brother and his father—and it just happened that there was an article on jelqing in Musclemag magazine that month. They both ended up trying it out. His father started because he married a woman 10 years younger than him, and cheerfully reports that his erections are "harder and stronger than ever."

The best part, Gary says, "I am not ashamed of my penis anymore. To me, performing penis exercises is like working out for your body, only for your dick. I feel good when I lift weights and run, and I feel good when I exercise my penis. It's not so much about getting bigger anymore for me. I feel like I'm big now. It's about improving myself in every way that I can—physically, mentally, emotionally, and spiritually. Penis exercising is just one little facet on my road of self improvement."

"I Built More than Just Inches in My Pants!"

Name: A.J. Alfaro
Online Alias: Big Al
Age: 33
Starting Size: Length 6.5", Girth 5"
Current Size: Length 8.5", Girth 6.5"

A.J. Alfaro has been involved in fitness and health since high school. "I used to read bodybuilding magazines and one thing that struck me was the inordinate number of ads for penis pumps and augmentation surgery," says Alfaro.

It wasn't long before the wheels started turning. "I knew that there was a better way to accomplish penis enlargement without the dangers, inconveniences, and overall unaesthetic effects of pumps or surgeries. From there, I set out to learn as much as I could about natural penis enlargement techniques. I have never received any complaints about my size, but what man wouldn't object to a couple of extra inches? So of course, I decided to use myself as a guinea pig."

The results: His penis is bigger and harder than ever. In less than six months, he gained 2 inches in length and 1.5 inches in girth. Once he reached his goal, Alfaro concentrated on stamina work. "Your penis can be too big, but it can never be too fit," he says.

Alfaro says the key to his success was a combination of lightly increasing the intensity every workout and obtaining proper rest. "You have to try and push the intensity a little further in order to produce gains," he says.

Alfaro couldn't be happier with his decision to be a lab rat for the rest of us. "It has definitely made me more confident in the bedroom! There is nothing like the look of shock and delight on a woman's face when she sees a very well endowed penis," he reports. "In that same vain, I have also found out that it is possible to be too big for some women! Thankfully, my wife is very pleased with my proportions."

But Alfaro's biggest success didn't come in the form of inches in his pants; it came in the form of helping others. Alfaro has spent a large part of the last 10 years helping spread the word about the great benefits of performing penis exercises. On his own account, he has helped over 250,000 men build the penis they want.

His best words of advice? "Any man thinking about performing penis exercises should consider the reasons why he wants to start." Chiefly, he says, "The main reason why any man should penis exercise should be because HE wants to change his penis—not to impress a particular woman."

"I Gained 3 Inches in Length and 1.5 Inches in Girth!"

Name: Dave
Online Alias: Jelktoid
Age: 54
Starting Size: Length 5.5", Girth 4. 5"
Current Size: Length 8.5", Girth 6"

Nothing is as painful as suspecting that your wife is cheating on you. For Jack, it was icing on the cake. He and his wife had numerous relationship problems at the time, and all of this amplified the slight insecurity he always had with his penis size.

"So one day I decided to see if the Internet contained any information about penis enlargement," says Jack. "I was surprised to find some credible information and I decided to give it a try. At that time, my penis was 5.5 inches erect length by 4.5 inches erect girth."

Jack knew enlarging his penis wouldn't fix the underlining problem with his marriage, but it would help in one area their relationship was lacking: sex.

"My wife later admitted to the affair and she told me that the guy had a large penis. This cemented my commitment to do what I could to increase my size," he says. "Sixteen months later, my penis is 8.5 inches erect and 6 inches girth. That's a gain of 3 inches of length and 1.5 inches of girth."

Jack cautions that it took time, dedication, and effort to reach his new size. "I have put a lot of hours into performing penis exercises," he says.

But for him, every hour was worth it. "I was able to mend my relationship with my wife, and we have since celebrated our 25th wedding anniversary."

"Due to my current size, increased confidence, and commitment, my wife has orgasms every time we have sex. There are even times when I am too large for her despite the fact that she has had three children."

For other men working towards a bigger penis, Jack recommends, "Try and develop a goal and a penis exercises plan. With all of the information that is available now, attaining higher levels of penis growth is indeed possible," he says. "Create a plan and dedicate sufficient time to do the regimen that you choose. Be dedicated. Don't waiver. Don't be afraid to try new techniques, but don't switch your routine constantly either."

"I Reached My Goal in a Little Over 3 Months!"

Name: Martin
Online Alias: Utopia
Age: 23
Starting Size: Length 6.7", Girth 4.35"
Current Size: Length 7.9", Girth 5.35"

When Martin was about to have sex, he'd have a hard time getting an erection—mostly because he was afraid of what the girl might think of him and his penis.

"I was insecure with my penis for many years. I use to feel that my penis was not big enough for my body, as I'm almost 2 meters tall . . . I've never had any complaints from a girl, but that didn't stop my insecurity from building up."

It didn't take long for Martin to start looking for alternative ways to enlarge his penis. After some searching, he learned of penis exercises. Shortly after, his gains rolled in rapidly. "In a little over 2 months, I gained 2 centimeters (0.8") in length and also 2 centimeters in girth. I was amazed, and people couldn't believe my story," he reports. "It was truly unbelievable, I was so excited that I took pictures to show anyone interested in penis exercises." After roughly three and a half months, he had verifiably gained an inch in both length and girth.

Martin largely accredits his success to his devotion. He never missed a workout. "The real trick," he says, "is to convince yourself that one missed workout will lead to the next. Skipping training—even every once in a while—will leave you with double amount the time needed, not to mention a bad feeling about yourself."

He also says his method of choosing a goal played a big role. Unlike most men—who set high goals right off the bat—Martin set small goals (in fractions of an inch), reached them, celebrated his progress, and then set a new goal. "That's how I stayed motivated."

The motivation paid off. "Through performing penis exercises, I changed my life," says Martin. "I don't feel insecure while having sex. I feel like I have total control of my life, and I can transform my penis just how I want. And if I can do it, anyone can!"

"Now I Believe!"

Name: Chris
Online Alias: Ophiosaurus
Age: 47
Starting Size: Length 5.5", Girth 4.5"
Current Size: Length 8", Girth 5.5"

Some guys start to feel insecure about their penis when a partner says a negative comment regarding their "manhood"; other guys have felt insecure about their penis for all of their post-adolescent life. The latter was the case for Chris.

"I knew I was smaller than average because I was athletic and saw a lot of naked guys in the dressing room and showers. I first became conscience of this fact when I was in 7th grade. But I had not gone through puberty yet and still had hope for my shriveled up acorn," says Chris. "I was a late bloomer and finally changes happened in the beginning of 11th grade. Man did I shoot up. I was over 6 feet tall. However, my dick forgot to get on the growth bus."

Statistically speaking, Chris was right around average. However, he felt that his penis should be more proportioned to his taller body frame. This led to downward spiral of insecurity. He hated going to the bathroom in public, he hated having to see a doctor if clothes were to be taken off, and he even feared death because he felt "they all would laugh in the morgue" (he laughs looking back on it now).

So Chris finally got to the point where he was fed up with his fears and decided to do something about it. "I got sick and tired of my small size over the years and was going to get a larger unit somehow," he says. He found penis exercises, and in two years he gained over 2 inches in length and 1 inch in girth. How did he do it? "It has been a long journey of hard work," he warns. "It was through sheer desire. Never give up, never quit. Work at it, work at it, work at it. You have to be committed and have the drive. You really have to want it and make performing penis exercises a daily part of your life."

Dan believes that if you have the commitment, you will reach your goal. How does he feel now that he's reached his? "All I can say is that it's awesome! My girlfriend is amazed and doesn't know what is going on but loves it. I got together with her when I was 6.5 inches in length and 5 inches in girth. She comes all the time now because I can reach places I couldn't before."

"Size does matter," says Chris. "I only wish I knew about penis enlargement years ago. I thought it wasn't possible without surgery. Now I believe."

"I Gained 4.5 Inches in Length and 1.5 Inches in Girth!"

Online Alias: Bib
Age: 50
Starting Size: Length 6", Girth 5"
Current Size: Length 10.5", Girth 6.5"

Bib started out at average—not too big, not too small, but not enough for him, either. When he learned of penis exercises back in 98' through a few websites, he thought it was all a crock. "I didn't believe any of it," he says. However, the websites seemed honest and made sense, so Bib went out on a limb—and gained a total of six inches over a period of three and a half years.

"I saw good early gains and things took off from there. I kind of got carried away and ended up performing penis exercises a lot more than I thought I would. But I like it," he reports. "I still can't believe it. When I pass a mirror naked and catch a glimpse, I still do a double take. Also, I catch my wife looking all the time, naked or clothed. She looks at my crotch more than my face. I also catch other women looking all the time (clothed of course)."

Bib accredits most of his length gains to hanging—an advanced form of stretching—and his girth gains to the uli exercise. But the most important part was how he increased the intensity: "baby steps. Each time I added weight, I did it in baby steps. In fact, it would be one step forward and one step back until I was not overwhelmed by the intensity."

Bib's wife didn't find out until the sixth or seventh month of the whole ordeal. He had to tell her—"the difference in sex was already very noticeable . . . She was already having much more powerful orgasms." By the time he reached 9 inches in length, his wife commented that it was long enough, but she wouldn't complain if he wanted more girth.

"My wife was fairly amazed at the increase. My penis has been the #1 topic of conversation for a long time and I don't always bring it up. She thinks penis exercises is analogous to women wanting larger breasts," says Bib. "She still talks about it, but seems more interested in using it. It is still a new toy. I almost never ask for sex. She always starts the proceedings."

"I Ignited a New Spark in My 40-Year Marriage!"

Name: Chuck
Online Alias: Dustpan
Age: 64
Starting Size: Length 5.25", Girth 3.75"
Current Size: Length 7.75", Girth 6"

Chuck always felt that he had a small penis. His less-than-average penis, however, never stopped him from being able to please his wife, so he never did anything about it. But eventually a problem far greater pushed Chuck over the edge: weak erections. At 62 years old, Chuck's erections weren't has hard as they use to be, and it was putting a damper on sex because he wasn't lasting long enough for his wife to climax.

So Chuck took matters into his own hands. He searched for an answer, and it came in the form of penis exercises. "The more I read about jelqing and stretching the more I believed it."

Chuck immediately noticed results. "Within the first month I could see some size change in length and girth. Even with the small amount that I had gained, I felt the difference in our sex life."

In less than three months, he gained 1.25 inches in length and .65 inches in girth, and his erections were stronger than ever. But Chuck didn't stop there. In roughly 18 months he completely remodeled his penis—gaining a total of 2.5 inches in length and 2.25 inches in girth. His penis is now four times bigger than what he started with.

The best improvement is in his sex life. "The other day the wife and I were talking about the difference between years ago and today's sex . . . and she said that it feels like she's a virgin all over again. With my larger penis she now has a harder and stronger climax than she ever had before . . . and my erections stay harder and last longer than ever. I also have a more explosive ejaculation than I ever had."

Chuck cautions that the results didn't happen overnight. He boosts his success largely on his solid work ethic and his dedication to increasing the intensity. "Penis enlargement takes time and commitment," says Chuck. "But every moment spent performing penis exercises has been worth it. Penis exercising has been a blessing for my wife and I—a new spark has pushed our marriage of 40 plus years to a new high!"

"I've Done More Than Improve My Penis!"

Name: Fredrick
Online Alias: Kingpole
Age: 45
Starting Size: Length 5.5", Girth 4.5"
Current Size: Length 8", Girth 6"

Many men start having erection problems when they reach their retirement years. Some men, like Fredrick, start having problems much earlier.

"I was only 36 years old when I started experiencing ED. I had been diagnosed with diabetes, which is one of the leading causes of erection issues." he says. "As a result, I lost over an inch in erect size and my flaccid penis shrank to less than two inches. It was difficult to urinate because I would piss on myself. It was embarrassing to say the least."

Fredrick's penis issues raged on for six years without a cure. Even worse, he had lost all sexual desire. "I was in medical assistant school, and women were approaching me and I felt horrible knowing that I could not give them what they wanted."

Then he learned of penis exercises. The exercises immediately started increasing his flaccid size, but the erection difficulties were so severe that it took several months to completely overcome. "Jelqing was the only way I could get an erection," he says.

The exercises were working, though, and it was all he needed to keep going. He was able to eventually obtain healthy, rock-hard erections. Within six months, he had gained over an inch in girth and nearly two inches in length. The whole experience felt surreal.

"When I first reached 6 inches in length, I was excited," he exclaims.

Then the unthinkable happened. He almost lost his life when his body started shutting down to a freak response to an antibiotic. It took a year and half and several hospital visits, but he was able to heal through a recovery program that involved natural supplements – all of which also helped his sexual health. He gradually started performing penis exercises again, and soon after the more gains followed.

"Now, I am at 8 inches in non-bone pressed length and over 6 inches in girth," Fredrick says.

For Fredrick, penis exercises have been more than way to improve his ED and penis size—although it's done that and much more. "Penis exercising has helped me when I've been in some really bad situations," he says. "I am now a Moderator on The PE Gym. I feel helping others get healthier is my thanks to God for healing me and putting the right people in my path to do so."

"Now I Enjoy a Much More Active Sex Life!"

Name: Bob
Online Alias: Going411by7
Age: 69
Starting Size: Length 7.75", Girth 5"
Current Size: Length 10.5", Girth 6"

Erection drugs are like a band-aide to hardness troubles: They help everything seem normal for a certain period of time, but they still leave the underlining issue intact. For Bob, enough was enough. He was sick of taking Viagra before sex and yearned for a long-term cure to his erection difficulties.

"I fell into penis exercises by accident," he says. "I was large to start with, so I was not looking to get a bigger dick. I was mainly looking to improve my erection quality."

He spent two months reading as much as he could about penis exercises—from routines that seemed to work best to the overall successes and failures of many men.

"One thing I learned is that you have to approach it as a long-term (for me a life-long) commitment," Bob says. "Some guys gain fast. Some don't. But like anything, you get out of it what you put into it. It's all about trial and error."

He gained a half inch the first couple of weeks, which motivated him to keep going. He also started waking up with a "massive rock-hard woody."

"I could not believe my eyes! It had been many years since I had experienced these kinds of erections," Bob says. "I was off to the races!"

Although he didn't gain the next two months, he continued to increase the length and intensity of his workouts. "This was where an act of faith came into play," he says. "I had this idea in my head that although I saw no further gains, that I would gain if I kept at it."

His act of faith worked. During the next several months, he started to gain rapidly—gaining an estimated 2 inches in erect length. Bob concludes that patience was the key ingredient to his success. "I eased myself into penis exercises. I started with a light jelqing and kegel routine so I wouldn't injure myself," he says. "This was paramount for me. I did not want to harm the only dick I had. I always stopped if there was any type of pain."

It's been five years since Bob started exercising his penis, and he's still at it just as strong as ever. "I know I have more energy now thanks to penis exercises, and my libido is incredibly strong for my age or for any age for that matter," he says. "Of course, I also now enjoy a much more active sex life and it's led to an all around improvement in my health."

"WOW, How Big is That Thing?"

Online Alias: PESG
Age: 20
Starting Size: Length 5.85", Girth 4.25"
Current Size: Length 8", Girth 5.75"

When couples fight, they can say rude things. When they break up, they can be blatantly cruel. The latter was the case for PESG.

"Apparently I had a small penis. Within weeks, the entire school knew that my member wasn't exactly the most endowed one on the planet," says PESG. "I became the laughingstock of the school by the female sex. I was borderline depressed."

In an attempt to change his penis size, PESG tried taking penis enlargement pills for several months. "I probably had some better blood flow but no changes in size," he says. "I started believing that there was no hope whatsoever."

Then he discovered penis exercises. "I started doing the exercises and I didn't stop. I was so determined that I never missed a session for three months," he says. "I didn't see incredible gains in the first 3 months, but I was growing bigger in both length and girth. My erection quality was also insane. With every passing month, my confidence grew more and more."

In two years, PESG gained 2.15 inches in erect length and 1.5 inches in erect girth. His flaccid size also increased by 2.2 inches. The best part? The routine he used to do it: 10 minutes of warming up, 10 minutes of jelqing and 10 minutes of stretching.

"For the first year, I did not change my routine one iota," says PESG. "My theory is why change what is working? If after three months I had good gains, then why change? Less really is better!"

Even more important than PESG's routine was his mindset. "I believe the three factors to successful penis enlargement are motivation, dedication, and perseverance," he says. "I believe you should also keep your dick at full flaccid as much as you can. Also, when it comes to masturbating and ejaculation, try to stay as close to the edge for as long as possible after a workout session. I personally release my load every third workout session."

How does PESG feel about the difference in his pants? His most recent sexual encounter says it all. "I just had sex with a girl who I know very well. Not only did I have three orgasms and our session lasted nearly two hours, but it also culminated with her saying 'WOW, how big is that thing?'"

"I Added Four Inches in Length and Two Inches in Girth!"

Name: John
Online Alias: JonPop
Age: 67
Starting Size: Length 4.75", Girth 4.25"
Current Size: Length 8.5", Girth 6.5"

Testosterone is a lifeline to overall growth, including penis growth. A deficiency of the hormone can lead to an underdeveloped penis, a lower sex drive, and a laundry list of other problems. For John, it was an issue that plagued him for most of his life. Due to a left testicle injury when he was 10 years old, he had a testosterone deficiency and wasn't able to fully develop his potential. He reports that his flaccid size was no bigger than a "button" and his erect length was a little over four and half inches.

"My dad was over eight inches and both my sons are huge," he says. "I always felt so cheated."

The good news? He was still able to maintain a healthy sex life. "I never had any complaints about my size from women, at least not to my face and I was with a lot of women before marriage."

The bad news? Taking a shower in the locker room with other men. "In school, I waited until everyone was done taking a shower before I took mine. . . but in the Army, I was forced to shower with everyone and I was teased and called, 'Needle Dick the Bug Fucker,'" said John. "This hurt deeply and I wound up in a lot of fights."

Notwithstanding, he married the love of his life and they've had a healthy relationship for many years. But he wanted more, and yearned to regain what he lost due to his testosterone deficiency. At age 60, his answer came in the form of penis exercises. His wife was supportive and, to her surprise, it worked. "My gains have been amazing," he says.

Along the way, he also fixed his testosterone issues. "My doctor did a blood test for testosterone and found that I was very low," says John. "He started me on testosterone injections on a 21 day cycle. This seemed to kick start my gains."

In a five year period, he has dramatically changed the look, size and feel of his penis – adding over two inches in girth and nearly four inches in length.

"It has increased our sex life dramatically. Not that it hasn't always been good, but I can't be anywhere in close proximity without her grabbing me around the neck for a hug and a bulge grab," he says. "Just yesterday, I was taking the clothes out of the dryer and she grabbed my penis and said, 'God, this thing is HUGE!' What a day that turned out to be."

"I Gained Confidence, Size, and Hardness!"

Name: Jake
Online Alias: Spruce
Age: 34
Starting Size: Length 5.5", Girth 4.75"
Current Size: Length 7", Girth 5.5"

Every man exercises his penis for a different reason. Jake had two. Reason 1: "Things had become very stale in my marriage. My wife didn't seem interested in sex anymore. I, as I usually do, assumed the problem might have been me, and I thought maybe I didn't have enough down there to excite her."

Reason 2: "What man doesn't want a bigger penis?"

Jake found the answer to his problems when he learned of penis exercises. He found out about jelqing and stretching through a free website. When he tried the exercises, the results poured in immediately.

Within three months, Jake gained nearly 1.5 inches in length and .75 inches in girth. "I attribute a lot of my gains to simply having a harder, healthier penis. I know when I started I didn't get the hard wood I am getting now."

While he doesn't do much penis exercise anymore, Jake has made a change—not only in his pants, but also in his thinking. "What I now realize is that my erect penis was always about average anyway. Even if I was below average, women were still attracted to me," he says. "I meet women now that I went to school with and find out they wanted me all along. Who would have ever thought? When I was younger, I spent so much time worrying about my damn penis I missed opportunities to use it."

"To the younger guys worrying about their size: just go for it. Be CONFIDENT and you will find that it really turns a woman on, regardless of your size."

Appendix F:

Survey Results: Does Ejaculating After a Penis Exercising Workout Influence Your Gains?

To masturbate or not to masturbate, that's the question.

We did an informal survey on PEGym.com asking community members about whether or not they masturbated within an hour after a normal penis exercising session. If they did, we wanted to know if they ejaculated. These results were then tied to gains, and the results were surprising.

Out of 542 respondents, 50 percent responded that they do masturbate within an hour of a penis exercising workout. In addition, most (76 percent) ejaculated during masturbation. The results were:

- 206 people answered yes they masturbate, and they ejaculate
- 65 people answered yest they masturbate, but they don't ejaculate
- 271 people answered no they don't masturbate within an hour of a penis exercising session

What was significant was the difference in enlargement results the men experienced in the three different responses.

- The men who answered "Yes and I ejaculate" showed the least amount of gains. Their overall penis size increase was 26.9 percent, with an average gain of 3.3 cubic inches.
- The men who answered "Yes and I do not ejaculate." reported an increase of 36.36 percent, with an average gain of 4.21 cubic inches.
- Lastly, the men who did not masturbate within an hour of performing penis exercises showed the most gains. The had an average increase of 37.6 percent in penis size, with an average gain of 4.52 cubic inches.

Although this informal survey showed that, on average, the respondents had increased their penis size by more than a third, masturbating within an hour, and even whether or not someone ejaculates when they masturbate within an hour of a penis exercising session, can impact your results. The men who did not masturbate experienced a significant size increase when compared to the men who did. Furthermore, from this study, it can be concluded that if you are going to masturbate within an hour of a penis exercising session, ejaculating can negatively impact your gains.

Appendix G:
Glossary

Adequate Rest: Obtaining adequate rest is one of the three principles in the "Circle of Gains" found in the penis enlargement book *Penis Exercises*. Obtaining rest while performing penis exercises is important as it allows your penis to heal and grow.

ADS (All Day Stretching Device): Common All Day Stretchers include extenders and light weights that hang from the penis. You can find the popular All Day Stretchers in our penis enlargement device directory.

Base: The base of the penis. Most often on this site, the base refers to the first visible part of the penis near the pubic bone. For example, *Encircle the* **base** *of your penis with an OK-grip.* However, anatomically speaking, the base of the penis is at the foundation of the inner penis, which is inside the body and above the perineum.

Body Clues: Body clues are the signs and symptoms your body gives you. Paying attention to your "body clues" is one of the three principles in the "Circle of Gains," found in the book *Penis Exercises*. Listening and following your body clues is absolutely vital to healthy and effective penis exercises.

Bone Pressed: To measure from pubic bone to the tip of the head, with the ruler pressed into the bone.

BPFSL (Bone Pressed Flaccid Stretched Length): Refers to a type of measuring of the flaccid penis. To measure BPFSL, stretch your flaccid penis out as far as possible (while it is in its stretchiest state, usually right after a warm up). Then measure from pubic bone to the tip of the head, with the ruler pressed into the bone.

BPEL (Bone Pressed Erect Length): Refers to a type of measuring: From pubic bone to the tip of the head, with the ruler pressed into the bone.

Bulbocavernosus Muscle: One of the chief pelvic floor muscles; also known as the BC muscle or the bulbospongiosus muscle. Along with assisting the process of erection, the bulbocavernosus muscle compresses the urethra, typically to empty it of residual semen or urine.

Bulbospongiosus Muscle: Another name for the bulbocavernosus muscle.

Cementing: Involves weaning yourself off a penis exercises routine in an effort to make your penis enlargement gains permanent.

Clamping Devices: Penis enlargement devices that work by clamping off the base of the penis, restricting blood flow and causing the penis to expand outward. See the Clamping 101 Advanced Penis Enlargement Guide.

COG (Circle of Gains): A termed coined in the penis enlargement book,*Penis Exercises*. The Circle of Gains is made of up the three essential principles of penis exercises: Obtain Adequate Rest, Gradually Increase the Intensity, and Watch Your "Body Clues."

Collagen: A protein that makes up the connective tissue within the penis.

Conditioning: Characterized by a penis that is highly adapted to penis exercises. Penis enlargement growth often slows down as result of being conditioned. Conditioning can often be undone by taking a long break to decondition the penis.

Corpora Cavernosa: The two top chambers of the penis; largely composed of collagen and smooth muscle. Hardens upon erection.

Corpora Spongiosum: The bottom of the penis; holds the urethra. Stays semi-soft upon erection.

Darkening Effect: Also known as discoloration. Darkening is a fairly common side effect that involves the penis, or parts of the penis, becoming darker.

Deconditioning: A break from penis exercises that reverses the effects of conditioning. An effective deconditioning break typically lasts six to twelve weeks.

Discoloration: See darkening effect.

Dry Jelq: To jelq without lubrication.

EG (Erect Girth): Most often refers to the erect girth measurement, which is in circumference. For example, My EG goal is 6 inches.

Ejaculate: To discharge semen.

Engorged: Filled with blood.

EQ (Erection Quality): A high or strong erection quality means you have "strong, firm and hard" erections. A weak or low erection quality means you have "weak, soft and not very hard" erections.

Erect Exercises: An intense form of penis exercises that involves the erect penis. Not advised for the at least six months, and definitely not for beginners.

Erectile Dysfunction: The inability to achieve or maintain an erection.

Erection Level: How engorged your penis is. The erection levels run from 0 to 100 percent and together make up the erection gauge. The higher your erection level, the more erect you are.

EVO (Essential Vein Oil): A penis exercises lubricant. EVO was created by a penis exerciser who uses the online alias Eroset.

Fat Pad: Refers to the fat that is positioned in front of your pubic bone. The smaller your fat pad, the more visible penis you have.

Flaccid: The state of the penis when it is not erect; soft; a zero percent erection level.

Frenulum: The slender strip of skin on the underside of the penis that joins the shaft to the head.

Glans: The head of the penis; the anatomical part of the penis where urine and semen are discharged.

Gradually Increase Intensity: *Gradually increase the intensity* is one of the three principles in the "Circle of Gains" found in the penis enlargement book, *Penis Exercises*. The keyword here is gradual, as many men up the intensity way before their penis is ready.

Grower: A man whose flaccid penis is small and dramatically grows upon erection. Opposite of a shower.

Intensity: The amount of force used; a measure of the amount of strength you are using when performing penis exercises.

Intensity Level: Helps you decipher how intense the exercise is. The higher the Intensity Level, the higher the intensity.

Ischiocavernosus Muscle: One of the chief pelvic floor muscles; also known as the IC muscle. The ischiocavernosus muscle contributes to erection by compressing the inner penis, which squeezes blood into the outer penis.

Jelq: A penis exercise that involves milking the blood throughout your penis. The jelq helps build penis length, girth, and hardness.

Jelq Device: A device that increases the intensity of your jelqs.

Kegel: An exercise that uses the pelvic floor muscles. The Kegel has an array of benefits, particularly increased hardness.

Manual Exercises: Penis exercises that use only the hands, opposed to exercises that use a penis enlargement device.

Mid Shaft: The middle of your penis; half way between your base and your glans.

Natural Penis Enlargement: The enlargement of the penis through penis exercises.

NBPEL (Non-Bone Pressed Erect Length): Refers to a type of measuring: To barely press the ruler against the skin when measuring length; not pressing the ruler into the pubic bone.

Nocturnal Erections: Random erections that take place during your sleep, most often in the REM stage of sleep.

Non-Bone Pressed: To barely press the ruler against the skin when measuring length; not pressing the ruler into the pubic bone.

Overhand Grip: Refers to the position of your grip, in which your fingers are facing the floor.

Over-training: Occurs when a man penis exercises more than his penis can handle. Over-training inhibits penis enlargement growth and leads to negative Physiological Indicators (PIs), such as weak erections.

PE: The acronym for one of the following, depending on the context: premature ejaculation, penis enlargement, or penis exercises. In the penis exercises community, PE most often stands for natural penis enlargement.

Penile: Of or relating to the penis.

Penis Enlargement: The enlargement of the penis. The most popular penis enlargement methods include penis exercises, the use of a device, and surgery. Our penis enlargement guide shows how to use penis exercises as a way for enlargement.

Penis Enlargement Device: A device designed to enlarge and exercise the penis.

Penis Exerciser: A man who penis exercises.

Penis Exercising: The act of exercising the penis.

Perineum: The region between the anus and testicles.

Petechiae: The medical name for spots that form on the penis. The spots are typically red and are fairly common in the beginning. They often occur due to jelqing.

Peyronie's Disease: Curvature of the penis caused by plaque formation inside the tunica. Peyronie's disease typically forms during adulthood and dissipates within one to two years.

Phallus: Of or relating to the penis.

Pincher Grip: A grip that forms a "pinching" hand gesture; places less pressure on the underside and the head of the penis. Looks as if you are *pinching* the penis.

Plateau: When penis enlargement gains come to a halt.

Point of No Return: The point in which semen starts moving through the urethra. Ejaculation is inevitable once you reach the point of no return.

Post-Micturition Dribble: A condition in which urine consistently dribbles from the penis at the end of an urination session.

Prostate: Refers to the prostate gland, which is an organ that encircles the urethra at the base of the bladder. The prostate gland controls the release of urine and secretes the alkaline fluid that holds semen upon ejaculation.

Pubic Bone: The bone that is located directly above your penis, right below your abdomen.

Pubococcygeus Muscle: A hammock-like muscle that extends from the pubic bone to the tailbone. Both males and females have a "PC" muscle.

Shaft: The main body of the penis.

Shock Routine: Penis exercising for several hours in one day in an effort to jump start penis enlargement gains or break a plateau. Shock routines are too intense for beginners. After a shock routine, you take a break for at least several days, and quite possibly a week or more.

Shower: A man whose penis is typically highly engorged and good for show (in accordance to size). A shower has a flaccid penis that doesn't grow much upon erection.

Skeletal Muscles: Striated muscles that are usually voluntary (smooth muscle is typically involuntary). Skeletal muscles include the biceps, quadriceps, abdomens, and other muscles. The pelvic floor muscles, located at the base of the inner penis, are skeletal muscles. You can strengthen these muscles and improve your sex life by using the Kegel.

SM (Smooth Muscle): Contrary to popular belief, the penis is roughly half muscle.

Sporadic Exercising: Randomly exercising the penis; following no specific routine.

Spotting: A moderately common side effect in the beginning in which spots (often red) form on the penis; medically known as petechiae.

Tunica: A strong, tendon-like tissue that covers the corpus chambers within the penis.

Urethra: The canal that semen and urine discharge from.

Urinary Incontinence: A condition that involves the involuntary excretion of urine, often in relation to another underlining medical condition. Urinary incontinence is more common in women than in men.

Urinate: To discharge urine; to go pee.

Vasodilator: A drug or nerve that opens the blood vessels and increases blood flow.

Warm Up: A method of heating the penis prior to performing penis exercises. A warm up increases probability of growth, decreases side effects, and decreases chances of injury.

Wet Jelq: To jelq with lubrication.

Afterword

"I enjoyed every inch of it."

-Mae West

It has been a pleasure to share the most up-to-date information that the penis exercises community has to offer. Make no mistake: the art of performing penis exercises is still in its infant stages and is constantly evolving. So if you're ever looking for more information, sign-in online. Go to http://www.PEGym.com or one of the highly recommended websites in Appendix D. There you will find more routines, exercises, and advice that will help you keep your penis fit and healthy for life. However, just as beneficial, you will find a community of men who yearn and love to improve themselves—and even greater—love to help other men.

Reference Notes

Chapter 1

1. According to a survey of the top 8 penis enlargement sites, their total members exceed 1.3 million men.
2. All the quotes in this book are taken directly from interviews or direct reports on forums such as ThundersPlace.com and PEGym.com

Chapter 2

1. Seidel, C.L., and N. W. Weisbrodt. *Hypertrophic Response in Smooth Muscle*. Boca Raton: CRC Press, 1987.
2. Kim, Y., et al. "Injection of Skeletal Muscle-Derived Cells into the Penis Improves Erectile Function." *International Journal of Impotence Research*. Vol. 18 (2006), pp. 329-324.
3. Wespes, E. "Smooth Muscle Pathology and Erectile Dysfunction." *International Journal of Impotence Research*. Vol. 14 (2002), pp. 17-21.

4. Aytac et al. estimated that 152 million men had erectile dysfunction in 1995 and that this number will increase to 322 million by 2025. Aytac, I.A., et al. "The Likely Worldwide Increase in Erectile Dysfunction Between 1995 and 2025 and Some Possible Policy Consequences." *British Journal of Urology International*. Vol. 84 (1999), pp 50-56.
5. Several doctors have done studies on the effects of a certain type of penis exercise known as the kegel, which works out the pelvic floor muscles. In one study conducted by Dr. Frank Sommer, urologist and professor at Hamburg University of Men's Health, kegels were more effective than erection drugs.
6. Many of these benefits have been reported by men in online support groups and forums, along with books and scientific journals like Dr. Grace Dorey's book. Dorey, Grace. *Pelvic Floor Exercises for Erectile Dysfunction*. London: Whurr Publishers, 2004.

Chapter 3

1. Kinsey, A. E. *Sexual Behavior in the Human Male*. Philadelphia: Saunders, 1948.
2. Wolf, Buck. "Are Men Getting Smaller Where It Counts? Recent Studies Revise Average Length of the Male Organ." ABC News. 2005.

Chapter 4

1. Zinczenko, D., Spiker, T. Men*, Love & Sex: The Complete User's Guide for Women*. New York: Rodale, 2006.
2. Griffin, Gary. *Penis Enlargement Methods—Fact & Phallusy*. Palm Springs: Added Dimensions, 1996.

Chapter 10

1. Curtis, Dan. *Dr. Dan's Super Weight Loss Plan*. Clearwater: Super Weight Loss Plan, 2005.

Chapter 13

1. Leech, Eric J., and Planet Green. "8 Vitamins and Herbs To Improve Your Sex Life Naturally." *TLC Cooking* . N.p., n.d. Web. 14 Jan. 2013. <http://recipes.howstuffworks.com/vitamins-herbs-sex-life.htm>.
2. "China-free Vitamin C Source." *The Vitamin C Foundation*. N.p., n.d. Web. 14 Jan. 2013. <http://www.vitamincfoundation.org/news.shtml>.
3. Venokur-Clark, Rachel. "Boost Your Libido With Vitamin B | Care2 Healthy Living." *Care2*. N.p., n.d. Web. 14 Jan. 2013. <http://www.care2.com/greenliving/boost-your-libido-with-vitamin-b.html>.

Chapter 14

1. Porter, Shane. "Sexual dysfunction: The escalating price of abusing porn.." *NSB News*. N.p., 12 Aug. 2012. Web. 14 Jan. 2013. <http://www.nsbnews.net/content/409829-sexual-dysfunction-escalating-price-abusing-porn>.
2. "Porn-Induced Sexual Dysfunction: A Growing Problem | Psychology Today." *Psychology Today*. N.p., n.d. Web. 14 Jan. 2013. <http://www.psychologytoday.com/blog/cupids-poisoned-arrow/201107/porn-induced-sexual-dysfunction-is-growing-problem>.

Chapter 15

1. Several of these benefits have been confirmed not only by men in online forums, but also by patients of sex therapists and by men in studies. Further references include: Chia, M., and D. Abrams. *The Multi-Orgasmic Man*. San Francisco: HarperCollins, 1996; Dorey, Grace. *Pelvic Floor Exercises for Erectile Dysfunction*. London: Whurr Publishers, 2004; Hsu, Geng-Long. "Hypothesis of Human Penile Anatomy." Asian Journal of Andrology. Vol. 8 (2006), pp. 225-234; Keesling, Barbara. *How to Make Love All Night*. New York:

HarperCollins, 1994; Kegel, Arnold H. "Stress Incontinence and Genital Relaxation; A Nonsurgical Method of Increasing the Tone of Sphincters and Their Supporting Structures." *Clinical Symposia*. Vol. 4. (1952), No. 2, pp. 35-51; Nixon, D., Gomez, M., *The Prostate Health Program*. New York: Simon and Schuster, 2004; Perry, J. D., and L. T. Hullet. *The Bastardization of Dr. Kegel's Exercise*. New Jersey: Northeaster Gerontological Society, 1988.

2. Dorey, Grace. *Pelvic Floor Exercises for Erectile Dysfunction*. London: Whurr Publishers, 2004.
3. Grace Dorey et al. "*Randomized* controlled trial of pelvic floor muscle exercises and manometric biofeedback for erectile dysfunction." *British Journal of General Practice*. Vol. 54 (Nov. 2004), pp. 819-25.

Chapter 26

1. The JAI stretch actually stands for Johan's Active Isolated stretch (Johan is the online alias of the man who discovered the exercise). Although active isolated stretches are meant for skeletal muscles and their tendons, many men have found that they work for penis exercises as well. As a side note, the uli and the horse squeeze are also named after the aliases of their creators.

Chapter 30

1. Ahmed Shafik, et al. "Electrophysiologic Activity of the Tunica Albuginea and Corpora Cavernosa: Possible Role of Tunica Albuginea in the Erectile Mechanism." *The Journal of Sexual Medicine*. Vol. 4 (2007), No.3, pp 675–679.

Chapter 33

1. Barlow, David H., Ali Mears, Dip Gum. *Sexually Transmitted Infections*. London: Oxford University Press, 2006.
2. Penile Mondor's disease is technically thrombosis of the main dorsal vein of the penis—the large vein that runs down the middle of the shaft. However, a recently published scientific article on penile

Mondor's disease suggests that all penile clotted, inflamed veins fall into the category of Mondor's—not just the dorsal vein. Technically this may not be the case, but the exact term of penile Mondor's is still a matter of debate in the scientific and medical communities. Other similar medical ailments that are often placed in the same category with penile Mondor's include sclerosing lymphangitis—inflammation of lymph vessels—and thromboses of smaller veins. Penile Mondor's disease references: Dicuio, M., et al. "Doppler Ultrasonography in a Young Patient With Penile Mondor's Disease." *Archivio Italiano di Urologia, Andrologia*. Vol. 77 (2005), No. 1, pp. 58-59; Griger, D.T., et al. "Penile Mondor's Disease in a 22-year-old Man" *The Journal of American Osteopathic Association*. Vol. 101 (2001), No. 4, pp. 235-237; Kraus, S., et al. "Mondor's Disease of the Penis." *Urologia Internationalis*. Vol. 64 (2000), No. 2, pp. 99-100; Kumarl, B., et al. "Mondor's Disease of Penis: a Forgotten Disease." *Sexually Transmitted Infections*. Vol. 81 (2005), No. 6, pp. 480-482; Ozkara, H., et al. "Superficial Dorsal Penile Vein Thrombosis (Penile Mondor's Disease)." *International Urology & Nephrology*. Vol. 28 (1996), No. 3. pp. 387-391; Sasso, F., et al. "Penile Mondors' Disease: an Underestimated Pathology." *British Journal of Urology*. Vol. 77 (1996), No. 5, pp. 729-732; Swierzewski, S.J. III, et al. "The Management of Penile Mondor's Phlebitis: Superficial Dorsal Penile Vein Thrombosis." *Journal of Urology*. Vol. 150 (1993), No. 1, pp. 77-78.

Appendices

1. Reinisch, June M. *The Kinsey Institute New Report on Sex*. New York: St. Martin's Press, 1991.
2. Dinsmore, W., Kell, P. *Impotence: A Guide for Men of All Ages*. London: RSM Press, 2002.
3. Chia, M., and D. Abrams. *The Multi-Orgasmic Man*. San Francisco: HarperCollins, 1996.
4. Keesling, Barbara. *How to Make Love All Night*. New York: HarperCollins, 1994.

5. Hays, Scott. *Built For Sex*. New York: Rodale, 2005; Kerner, Ian. He Comes Next. New York: HarperCollins, 2006; Klotz, T., et al. "Effectiveness of Oral L-Arginine in First-Line Treatment of Erectile Dysfunction in a Controlled Crossover Study." Urologia Internationalis. Vol. 63 (1999), No. 4, pp. 220-223; Lamm, Steven. The Hardness Factor. New York: HarperCollins, 2005.
6. The pictures used for the devices are of a DustPan Hanger, Penis Exercise Weights, a PenisMaster, extender, a FastSize extender, a Jelq Device, an LA Pump, and a Cable Clamp.
7. On the TV show *The View*, Dr. Steven Lamm mentioned extenders can help cure Peyronie's disease.
8. Keesling, B. (19971993). *Making love better than ever: how to increase your sexual pleasure*. London: Piatkus.
9. Howard II, D. R. (2012, August 2). The Precise Mechanism of the Penis Enlargement Response through Manual and Mechanical Intervention. *The PE Gym*. http://www.pegym.com/articles/precise-mechanism-pe-response-manual-mechanical-intervention
10. Berk, Bradford C. "Vascular Smooth Muscle Growth: Autocrine Growth Mechanisms." Physiological Reviews. Vol. 81 (2001), No. 3, pp. 999-1030. Christ, George J. "The Penis as a Vascular Organ." *Urologic Clinics of North America*. Vol. 22 (1995), No. 4, pp. 727-745; Cohen, Joseph. The Penis Book. New York: Broadway Books, 2004; Costa, W. S., et al. "Comparative Analysis of the Penis Corpora Cavernosa in Controls and Patients with Erectile Dysfunction." BJU International. Vol. (2006), pp. 567-569; Dorey, Grace. *Pelvic Floor Exercises for Erectile Dysfunction*. London: Whurr, 2004; Kiviat, M. D., et al. "Smooth Muscle Regeneration in the Ureter. Electron Microscopic and Autoradiographic Observations." American Journal of Pathology. Vol. 72 (1973), No. 3, pp. 403-416; Li, Chi-Ying, et al. "Penile Suspensory Ligament Division for Penile Augmentation: Indications and Results." *European Urology*. Vol. 49 (2006), No. 4, pp. 729-733; Moore, M., and C. Costa. *Dick: A User's Guide*. New York: Marlowe & Company, 2003; Schultzcu, Louis R. *Out in the Open: The Complete Male Pelvis*. California: North Atlantic Books,

1999; Seidel, C.L., and N. W. Weisbrodt. *Hypertrophic Response in Smooth Muscle.* Boca Raton: CRC Press, 1987; Sutton, Amy L. *Back and Neck Sourcebook.* Omnigraphics, second edition, 2004.

11. Eroset originally posted the instructions online at *ThundersPlace.com.* The instructions were printed with his permission.
12. Only 684 men were used in this average gains assessment—opposed to all 957 men who were surveyed—because not every man who took the survey answered the appropriate questions for the assessment.
13. The quotes in the success stories came from a combination of interviews and reports on forums (most notably *ThundersPlace.com*).

Index

Basic stretch, 27, 28, 53, 73, 89, 90, 92, 93, 94, 148, 155, 178
Body clues, 22, 31, 37, 38, 39, 40, 52, 91, 109, 110, 111, 112, 113, 114, 116, 120, 123, 127, 129, 136, 140, 141, 142, 146, 149, 150, 155, 158, 173, 195, 215, 272, 273
Body clues cheat sheet, 38
Caffeine, 196
Cementing, 11, 20, 28, 105, 141, 143, 166, 169, 170, 171, 172, 173, 273
Cool down, 69, 70, 118
Curved penis, 176
Darkening effect, 42, 65, 124, 125, 126, 127, 129, 142, 191, 274
Doughnut effect, 42, 123, 130, 142
Dry jelq, 85, 86, 87, 126, 131, 274
Ejaculating (before or after a workout), 115, 116, 201, 245, 270, 271
Ejaculation
    Further shooting distance of, 12, 55
Erectile dysfunction
    Due to over-training (temporary), 64, 123, 135, 136, 138, 142, 149
Erectile dysfunction, 7, 11, 39, 45, 49, 50, 51, 55, 57, 64, 123, 133, 135, 136, 137, 138, 142, 149, 208, 274
Erection difficulties
    Supplements for, 45, 136, 183, 184, 196
Erection level gauge, 78, 79, 80, 215, 274
Grower, 81, 197, 275
Intensity, 12, 28, 31, 35, 36, 37, 39, 40, 42, 52, 55, 81, 97, 98, 99, 101, 104, 110, 111, 112, 113, 115, 116, 119, 120, 121, 125, 127, 129, 132, 133, 134, 137, 138, 141, 142, 143, 146, 148, 149, 150, 151, 152, 155, 158,

Intensity (cont.), 163, 164, 171, 173, 175, 185, 189, 245, 255, 256, 261, 263, 265, 273, 275
Intensity levels, 148, 149, 173, 175, 274
JAI stretches, 93, 94, 118, 158
Jelq
How to, 53, 73, 74, 75, 76, 78, 80, 81, 82, 83, 84, 85, 86, 95, 121, 155
Mini jelq, 179
Origin of, 75, 76
Side jelq, 155, 177, 178, 179, 221
Vertical jelq, 155, 179, 222
Without lubrication, 85, 86, 87, 126, 131, 274
Kegel
Erectile dysfunction, 55, 57
How to, 28, 54, 55, 56, 57, 59, 60, 61, 62, 215, 216
Over-training, 63, 64
Premature ejaculation, 55, 56, 62, 64, 179, 198, 199
Reverse kegels, 62, 199, 200, 203
Masturbation, 10, 34, 50, 51, 75, 96, 108, 115, 130, 132, 135, 136, 137, 138, 202, 204, 245, 270
Morning wood, 38, 39
Multiple orgasms, 12, 55, 180
Muscle, 5, 6, 7, 8, 10, 11, 20, 27, 28, 33, 35, 36, 38, 42, 55, 56, 57, 58, 59, 60, 61, 62, 63, 64, 67, 75, 94, 98, 116, 128, 136, 145, 152, 153, 156, 166, 171, 179, 180. 181, 185, 199, 200, 201, 204, 206, 207, 208, 209, 211, 255, 274, 275, 277, 279, 280
Nocturnal erection, 10, 276
OK-grip, 75, 83, 85, 86, 272
Over-training, 11, 31, 36, 38, 39, 40, 42, 60, 64, 74, 102, 103, 109, 112, 113, 119, 124, 136, 137, 138, 139, 142, 149, 158, 166, 170, 181, 252, 276
Pain, 3, 38, 67. 90, 116, 117, 123, 124, 128, 133, 135, 176, 177, 198, 199, 200, 265
Penile Mondor's Disease, 123, 133, 134, 135, 190, 248

Penis enlargement
Devices, 28, 29, 70, 86, 125, 131, 134, 153, 167, 175, 186, 187, 188, 189, 190, 191, 192, 193, 197, 198, 209, 249, 250, 273, 274, 277, 278
Pills, 184, 185, 266
Surgery, 187, 191, 193, 194, 210, 256, 260, 276
Permanent gains. See Cementing,
Peyronie's disease, 177, 189, 208, 277
Pincher grip, 85, 86, 87, 128, 130, 179, 277
Plateau, 36, 118, 144, 145, 147, 158, 163, 164, 165, 166, 167, 168, 187, 277
Pornography, 13, 47, 48, 49, 50, 51, 52
Premature ejaculation
Fix and have multiple orgasms, 12, 55, 179, 180
How to fix. See Kegel
Prostate, 12, 55, 58, 63, 132, 201, 207, 277
Rest, 30, 31, 33, 34, 37, 39, 40, 52, 60, 64, 73, 111, 112, 113, 115, 119, 120, 132, 136, 137, 155, 158, 163, 167, 175, 185, 191, 256, 272, 273
Routines
Alternate, 162
Basic advancing routine, 114, 154, 158, 173
Basic beginner's, 97, 98, 99, 100, 101, 102, 103, 104, 106, 107, 108, 109, 111, 113, 141, 142, 154
Cementing, 11, 20, 28, 105, 141, 143, 166, 169, 170, 171, 172, 173, 273
Least work/max gain (advanced), 160
Least work/max gain (beginner), 103, 104, 105, 142, 174
Plateau-Breaking "shock workout," 163, 164, 167, 277
Progressive (advanced), 159
Progressive (beginner), 101, 102, 142

Split, 161

Shower, 81, 195, 197, 275, 277

Side effects

- Causes, 124, 125, 126, 127, 128, 129, 130, 131, 132, 133, 134, 136, 137
- Common, 21, 41, 42, 132, 274, 276
- Uncommon, 142
- What to do, 123, 125, 127, 129, 130, 131, 132, 135, 136

Smoking, 44, 186

Spots, 42, 65, 123, 125, 128, 129, 130, 142, 276, 278

Thrombosis. See Penile Mondor's Disease.

Turtle/Turtling effect, 66, 129, 196, 197, 198

Veins, 42, 76, 133, 134, 135, 196, 206, 207, 208

Acknowledgments

To the wonderful men and women that make up the “penis enlargement” community at the PEGym.com. This book wouldn’t have been possible without the collaboration of many men working towards decoding the “holy grail” of penis exercises.

- Thank you to ThunderSS, and http://www.thundersplace.com, for his generosity toward all men (regardless if they have a credit card or not).
- A particular special thank you to the men who helped shape our penis exercises beliefs and helped form this book either directly or indirectly, especially the men who use the following aliases: avocet8, babbis, BBS, Bib, Big Girtha, Bird2, BTC, Dino9x7, DLD, Dustpan, Eroset, Higherone, hobby, Merlin, ModestoMan, Mr. Happy, Para-Goomba, peforeal, penismith, Peter Dick, RedZulu2003, Shiver, sparkyx, stillwantmore, the “m” brothers—mbuc and mgus, ‘The Programmer’, Wadzilla (along with the kitchen sink and his big gainer friend), westla “Masturbation Doesn’t Affect Gains” 90069. You guys keep the penis exercises community running at full speed ahead.
- To the men who kindly allowed us to interview, question, and quote them in this book.
- To “Sparkyx” for his diligent work and keen thinking on discovering the physiological indicators (known as “body clues” in this book).

- To Brad and Brian from FastSize for their hard work on getting more medical backing for penis exercises.

- To Dr. Richard Howard for his continual support, persistent advice, and endless supply of information.

- To the moderators and contributors of The PE Gym for keeping the community in stride: Banana, Big Al, calixto, Cernunnos, Dance Sucka, Dustpan, going411by7, GTO, Hairtrigger, Iguana, imac, jayhawk11, JonPop, kingpole, Larger, newleo, PEsuccessGuy, Radiohead, ReetB, Rockitman, ronnierokk, SweetyV22, vegetarian, Waylander, W.M.P., whyleo, and the rest! You gentlemen are at the front lines of helping our fellow man in immeasurable ways.

- To my nameless and faceless model. Your dedication is more than admirable. It took months and hundreds upon hundreds of correspondences, but every step was well-spent and enjoyable.

Endnote

The information in this book is provided for general medical information purposes only and is not a guide on what you should do. It is only a collection of what other men have done. This book does not replace the advice of a medical professional. Please consult your physician for diagnostic and treatment options pertaining to your specific medical condition(s).

CPSIA information can be obtained
at www.ICGtesting.com
Printed in the USA
LVOW04s0225160516
488414LV00023B/426/P